Palgrave Studies in the History of Childhood

Series Editors
George Rousseau
University of Oxford, UK

Laurence Brockliss
University of Oxford, UK

Palgrave Studies in the History of Childhood is the first of its kind to historicise childhood in the English-speaking world; at present no historical series on children/childhood exists, despite burgeoning areas within Child Studies. The series aims to act both as a forum for publishing works in the history of childhood and a mechanism for consolidating the identity and attraction of the new discipline.

More information about this series at
http://www.palgrave.com/gp/series/14586

Lynne Curry

# Religion, Law, and the Medical Neglect of Children in the United States, 1870–2000

## 'The Science of the Age'

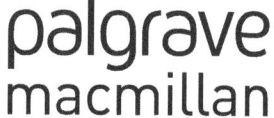

palgrave
macmillan

Lynne Curry
Eastern Illinois University
Charleston, IL, USA

Palgrave Studies in the History of Childhood
ISBN 978-3-030-24691-4     ISBN 978-3-030-24689-1   (eBook)
https://doi.org/10.1007/978-3-030-24689-1

Cover credit: Photo Josse/Leemage/Contributor

This Palgrave Macmillan imprint is published by the registered company Springer Nature
Switzerland AG
The registered company address is: Gewerbestrasse 11, 6330 Cham, Switzerland

*For Brandon*

# ACKNOWLEDGEMENTS

Historians acquire many debts in the process of pursuing long-term projects, and I am certainly no exception. I am especially grateful to George Rousseau and Laurence Brockliss, Series Editors of the *Palgrave Studies in the History of Childhood*, for including my work in their prestigious series. Emily Russell was the epitome of professionalism and courtesy, smoothing the way through the long and complex process that brings a historian's labors to fruition. I would like to thank Eastern Illinois University for providing me with professional support in the form of a sabbatical leave, arriving just in time as many years of research finally began to coalesce into something resembling a coherent historical monograph. Less formal, but no less valuable, support was given to me by my colleagues in the History Department who patiently read and commented on several pieces of this project at various and sundry stages of its evolution at our department's congenial colloquiums. A significant number of librarians and archivists guided my research over the years, a long list that includes the highly professional staffs at Booth Library at Eastern Illinois University, the University of Illinois College of Law, Styberg Library at the Garrett-Evangelical Theological Seminary, and the Zion-Benton Public Library. I wish to especially thank Kurt Morris at the Research and Reference Services at the Mary Baker Eddy Library for granting me access to their rich and invaluable collections as well as the staff who assisted me there. The cheerful docents of the Zion Historical Society allowed me to roam freely through Shiloh House, the residence of John Alexander Dowie, one extremely cold winter's afternoon.

The historical picture that eventually emerged from my research was significantly enriched through critiques and suggestions offered in a variety of venues, including academic conferences sponsored by the Society for the Social History of Medicine, King's College London, Université d'Angers, and San Francisco State University. At its later stages my work benefited greatly from insights offered by James Marten, Robert D. Johnston, and the anonymous reviewers at Palgrave Macmillan. A final and heartfelt word of thanks goes to my family and friends who have urged me onward, none more so than my husband Brandon who has read every word of this book and offered his careful thoughts, as a supportive partner as well as a clear-eyed scientist.

# CONTENTS

# CHAPTER 1

# Introduction

In the early twentieth century, controversies erupted when the children of parents who rejected scientific medicine as a tenet of their faith died of medically treatable conditions. Criminal trials brought parents' decisions in caring for their little ones under the glare of public scrutiny, and the fraught discourses that surrounded them shifted concerns about children's physical welfare beyond the walls of the private household. Throughout the remainder of the century, medical neglect cases rendered the bodies of children into sites of contention as broader medical and legal developments converged, and indeed collided, to produce these periodic controversies. This book examines religious-based medical neglect as a historical phenomenon that reflects changing social constructions of childhood in the United States.

By the last decades of the nineteenth century, an evolving understanding of children as distinct beings with particularized needs for physical care had begun to inform a broad spectrum of thinking well beyond the medical school lecture hall. The specialty of pediatrics emerged in the 1880s and evolved over the following decades in tandem with a vigorous child welfare movement that brought unprecedented public attention to matters concerning children's physical well-being. As medical historians Alexandra Minna Stern and Howard Markel have noted, campaigns to improve children's health rendered infant and childhood mortality rates into gauges

© The Author(s) 2019
L. Curry, *Religion, Law, and the Medical Neglect
of Children in the United States, 1870–2000,*
Palgrave Studies in the History of Childhood,
https://doi.org/10.1007/978-3-030-24689-1_1

by which to measure the nation's social progress. The new laboratory sciences, particularly bacteriology, revolutionized the theory and practice of public health and held out the promise that a range of deadly childhood diseases could be conquered if responsible adults became informed about, and assiduously followed, the precepts of scientific medicine. Advocates of the "new public health" urged modifications in children's immediate environments while physicians urged parents, particularly mothers, to monitor their children's bodies closely, remaining alert to any signs indicating possible dangers and seeking out the services of trained and licensed medical practitioners should a child's illness require professional intervention. Among the most dramatic developments of the era was the identification of *Corynebacterium diphtheriae* as the cause of diphtheria in 1884 by bacteriologists Edwin Klebs and Friedrich Löffler, followed by the discovery of diphtheria antitoxin by Emil von Behring in 1901. These breakthroughs occurring in German laboratories came at a time when diphtheria was a leading cause of death for American children under the age of fourteen. Historian Evelynn Maxine Hammonds has argued that the success of early twentieth-century campaigns to control the childhood scourge of diphtheria marked a critical moment in securing broader social authority for practitioners of scientific medicine in the United States. Not surprisingly, then, some of the earliest religious-based medical neglect controversies involved parents' refusal to secure diphtheria antitoxin for their children who were infected with the disease.[1]

An increasingly medicalized view of children's welfare also found its way into American law, as courts and legislatures re-examined adults' duties in light of changing understandings of children's needs for physical care. Legal scholar David S. Tanenhaus has argued that the decades following the Civil War saw courts and lawmakers struggling to balance a notion of children as autonomous actors endowed with rights of their own with their status as vulnerable and dependent beings whose very survival depended upon the protection of the state. Long-established legal doctrines had obligated adults to provide the life-sustaining necessities of food, clothing, and shelter to the children living under their care. A fourth category of necessity was "physic," a general and rather vague reference to the treatment of illness and injury. Throughout much of the nineteenth century parents had enjoyed an array of choices in meeting this obligation, as a variety of medical sects flourished and folk healing wisdom, supplemented with instructions from popular domestic advice manuals, informed adults' decisions in caring for children's health. In the century's last decades, however, the term "medical attendance" began to replace the archaic "physic" in both statutory language and legal discourse, and courts began to hold adults to more exacting standards in providing for children's physical care. At the same time, states were raising their education and training requirements for licensing the practice of medicine and, in many cases, prohibiting alternative practitioners such as homeopaths, hydropaths, and botanical healers from advertising themselves as medical doctors. Thus by the end of the nineteenth century, the legal requirement to provide medical attendance to a sick or injured child came to mean securing the services of licensed "regular" or mainstream physicians. Failure to provide professional medical attendance for conditions now regarded as treatable became defined as neglect within newly enacted child endangerment statutes. A few states went further, pursuing charges of manslaughter against parents whose children died of preventable causes without receiving medical attention. But, while scientific medicine held out great promise for saving children's lives, it could offer no hard-and-fast guarantees and, as tragic incidents in which children died due to contaminated smallpox vaccines and diphtheria antitoxin made clear, its use could cause harm as well as healing. Parents who rejected mainstream medicine pointed to the ongoing uncertainties of science in arguing that their choices placed neither their children's health nor their lives at risk. Christian Scientists in particular insisted that they did not, in fact, neglect their sick and injured children because they employed the services of metaphysical healers who were trained and certified by their church. Given the ambiguities of scientific medicine, courts struggled to establish bright-line standards for determining adults' legal obligations in providing medical care to children.[2]

Despite the optimism that medical advances inspired, many Americans remained wary of treading too far on the prerogatives that parents had traditionally enjoyed to raise their children as they saw fit. The emergence and rapid growth of new healing religions in the last half of the nineteenth century reflected an underlying uneasiness toward the growing presence of science in American life. Historian T. J. Jackson Lears has argued that antimodernist movements in this period represented a reaction against the rapid acceleration of industrial and urban growth that followed the Civil War. In the 1870s the influential Chicago-based evangelist Dwight L. Moody preached that the precepts of modern science, especially Darwinism's depiction of evolutionary change as the result of indiscriminate natural selection rather than the guiding hand of a loving God, alienated traditional communities and debased the values of modern life. Biographer

Stephen Gottschalk posited that the founder of Christian Science, Mary Baker Eddy, envisioned the church she established in 1879 as the vanguard of a counter-revolution against the "scientific materialism" that had begun to permeate American society. For Eddy, the belief that human beings were both physical and mortal had been reversed by the resurrection of Jesus, an eternal and unchanging truth that had been revealed in scripture but subsequently forgotten by Christians through the ages. The metaphysical healing system upon which Christian Science was founded sought to demonstrate that physical illness, and even death itself, was merely illusory. Stories of successful cures, widely circulated in the *Christian Science Journal*, enabled Eddy's church to become the fastest-growing of the new healing religions, attracting adherents throughout the United States. John Alexander Dowie, who in 1896 diverged from the divine healing movement to establish the Christian Catholic Church in Chicago, declared nothing less than a "holy war" against physicians in that city insisting that, while God alone possessed the power to heal the sick and injured, he had been blessed with the gift of channeling that power through the medium of his own hands. Dowie's publication *Leaves of Healing* prominently featured stories of miraculous cures, many involving children, attracting worried parents of sick and injured children well beyond the city of Chicago to the divine healer's activities. Many of those who were drawn to the new healing religions objected to scientific medicine's privileging of physical over spiritual concerns in child-rearing and worried that the growing social influence of medical doctors undermined parental authority in the home. They also pushed back against the incursion of the state into family matters traditionally circumscribed within the private household. Supporters of spiritual healing insisted that parents' choice to reject scientific medicine as a tenet of their faith represented the free exercise of religion and thus it must enjoy legal protection as a right delineated in the First Amendment to the United States Constitution.[3]

Many faiths, of course, regard science and prayer as complementary, rather than competing, contributors to the healing process. The theme of healing, as Amanda Porterfield has pointed out, is integrally threaded throughout ritual practices and theological precepts that are central to Christianity. In the nineteenth century a number of medical sects, including homeopathy, osteopathy and the variety of practices known as "magnetic" healing, had distinctly metaphysical dimensions that attributed health and illness to obscure forces operating beyond the limits of the physical world. Seventh-day Adventist founder Ellen G. White worked closely with John

Harvey Kellogg, a physician and health reformer who headed the highly regarded Battle Creek Sanitarium, and periodically revised her church's doctrines to comport with new understandings of bodily health and illness that emerged from mainstream medical science. Historian Heather D. Curtis has shown that participants in the mid-nineteenth century's divine healing movement regularly debated the question of which bodily conditions counted as sickness and differed over when the resort to medical remedies was acceptable to the faith. Two of spiritual healing's most influential leaders, however, urged their followers to make an unequivocal choice between scientific medicine and spiritual healing. Both Mary Baker Eddy and John Alexander Dowie employed aggressive rhetoric that framed the choice between spiritual and secular healing in stark and belligerent terms, creating a profound dilemma for devout parents whose children became ill or injured. Many sincere believers endured intense physical pain themselves, or allowed their children to suffer, as a sign of their steadfast commitment to these leaders' teachings.

A historical examination of religious-based medical neglect controversies reveals a more complex narrative than a reductive "science versus religion" model might suggest. Some of the new healing churches' most vociferous critics were in fact mainline Protestant clergy who warned their congregations against radical faith healing practices that eschewed all forms of medical attendance, especially when those being denied care were children too young or too ill to seek help of their own accord. Nor did proponents of religious healing always present a united front against their secular detractors. Dowie regularly denounced Christian Science as "mere mesmerism," while Eddy herself took to the courts to protect her proprietary interests from competitors whom she believed had appropriated and distorted her healing system. Both Dowie and Eddy, in fact, maintained a complex relationship with scientific medicine, adopting the title of doctor for themselves at various times in their careers even as they denounced mainstream or "regular" physicians. While he was a divinity student and hospital chaplain at the University of Edinburgh, Dowie had been exposed to instruction at the premier center of western medical education, and he drew upon that experience both to assert his own status as the social equal of licensed physicians in the United States and to denounce the depraved and barbaric practices he claimed to have witnessed in Edinburgh's anatomy laboratories. In 1881 Eddy founded the Massachusetts Metaphysical College in Boston as a state-chartered institution to train and credential practitioners of her own distinctive healing system. Eddy listed herself as a Professor of Obstetrics in the college's literature as well as in some early editions of her church's foundational text, *Science and Health with Key to the Scriptures*. Despite their attacks on the inefficacies and falsehoods of mainstream medicine both leaders frequently drew upon physicians' emerging social authority to provide scientific verification that bodily healing had taken place by spiritual means, authentications that regularly appeared in official publications and broadcast their churches' success stories well beyond their respective headquarters. Finally, despite their confrontational rhetoric Dowie and Eddy each made compromises with scientific medicine and its practitioners when exigent legal and personal circumstances moved them to do so.[4]

Mainstream medicine's response to practitioners of alternative forms of health care was frequently hostile, particularly as the American Medical Association moved to consolidate regular physicians' dominance over their competitors in the medical marketplace. Nevertheless, the late nineteenth-century's surge of interest in spiritual healing in the United States resists easy characterization solely as a populist revolt against professional elites and medical monopolies. Historian Michael C. Willrich has traced the complex social and intellectual origins of a robust movement that arose in reaction to compulsory vaccination measures imposed by health authorities in a number of states when smallpox epidemics hit major cities. While followers of spiritual healers were often denounced as ignorant and gullible rubes in big city newspapers and professional medical journals, many of those attracted to the new healing churches were in fact educated, lived in urban areas, and fell along a spectrum of socioeconomic classes. Founded in New England the First Church of Christ, Scientist shared a direct cultural heritage with the secular intellectual movement known as New Thought, a background clearly reflected in the membership of Eddy's church, which included a large proportion of white, middle-class, and professional congregants, a significant proportion of whom were female. On the other hand, it was often ordinary Americans rather than over-zealous public health officials or politically powerful doctors who sought help from police, legislators, and courts when they feared people were suffering needlessly without mainstream medical attendance, particularly when the untreated victims were vulnerable women and children. Neighbors complained to local health authorities when contagious disease cases went unreported and alerted coroners' offices when suspect deaths occurred under faith healers' care.[5]

As the twentieth century progressed, and the early promise of bacteriology began to be fulfilled through a number of preventive and therapeutic innovations, the clear benefits of scientific medicine to children's physical welfare could be more clearly discerned. After World War II physicians, particularly pediatricians, became dominant cultural voices in child-rearing, reaching millions of American households through the expert advice they proffered in popular books, mass circulation magazines, radio broadcasts, and television programs. In the 1960s, pediatricians took a leading public role in renewing the national discourse surrounding child abuse and neglect, arguing that their special medical expertise placed them in a unique position to diagnose cases of adult violence perpetrated against children and pressing for new laws requiring medical professionals to report suspected cases to child protective authorities. Fearing that an increasingly medicalized view of children's welfare weakened societal support for religious healing, supporters turned their attention to securing special exemptions for their practices within states' child abuse and neglect laws. By the mid-twentieth century, Christian Scientists already had been successful in gaining religious exceptions within a range of statutes pertaining to public health regulations and the licensing of medical practitioners. Church officials now took a leading role in lobbying for the insertion of statutory language to clarify that parents' choices to rely exclusively on religious healing would not be defined as child endangerment. The trend reached the federal level when religious exemptions found their way into administrative rules pertaining to the Child Abuse and Prevention Treatment Act of 1974 and the Parental Rights and Responsibilities Act passed by Congress in 1995. Opponents of religious exemptions argued that legal protections for adults who eschewed scientific medical care were responsible for the tragically unnecessary deaths of children from preventable causes. Today, while the nature and scope of laws vary across the United States, all but six states allow some form of religious exemption to the legal duty to provide medical attendance to a sick or injured child. The topic recently has gained a renewed sense of urgency as outbreaks of childhood diseases such as pertussis and measles, widely regarded as relics of a benighted past, have once again caught the public's attention and prompted physicians such as Paul A. Offit to call for the repeal of religious exemptions for mandatory childhood immunizations.[6]

Numerous legal scholars have explored pressing questions about children's right to equal protection under the law that are raised by the persistence of religious exemptions in child abuse and neglect laws, a status quo that distinguishes the United States from most other countries today. Martha Albertson Fineman reminds us that, historically, Americans' understandings of the family have been shaped by particular religious doctrines that defined a "natural" family unit and linked individuals' legal rights and responsibilities to membership within that unit. This deep-seated historical foundation is reflected in Americans' present-day unwillingness to embrace the human rights orientation of the United Nations' Convention on the Rights of the Child, an international treaty the United States has not ratified. Barbara Bennett Woodhouse has traced the historical antecedents of ongoing theoretical tensions between acknowledging children's rights that are "needs-based," such as having adequate food and clothing, and accepting those that are "capacity-based," such as the right to due process in legal proceedings. By contrast, scholars have been less engaged in exploring the emergence and evolution of the concept of medical neglect as a reflection of broader historical developments occurring in the nineteenth and twentieth centuries. Rennie B. Schoepflin, Shawn Francis Peters, and Alan Rogers have made important and insightful contributions to our understanding by placing highly contested, and disturbing, religious-based medical neglect cases under the historian's analytical lens.[7]

My aim is to shift the focus of this inquiry so that the history of childhood appears at the center of the historical picture. In her pathbreaking study of lawsuits involving the accidental deaths of children at the turn of the twentieth century, sociologist Vivian A. Zelizer uncovered a profound societal shift as children came to be regarded as economically "useless" but emotionally "priceless" to their parents. Similarly, historians examining the period 1870–1930 have traced the manifestation of changing societal attitudes concerning children's physical welfare in the appearance of legal battles to combat industrial, domestic, and sexual violence against children. Nevertheless, as Linda Gordon's work has made clear, many historical efforts at "rescuing" children perceived to be at physical peril did not meet with unqualified success, particularly when they were framed as contests between the interests of children and their parents. While deaths due to religious-based medical neglect have occurred very rarely in the United States, I argue that the first legal prosecutions of parents, and the controversies that surrounded them, signaled an epistemic shift in Americans' thinking about children as discrete biological beings with specialized needs for physical care. Supported by a broad child welfare movement that asserted the physical well-being of children as a matter of national interest, medical neglect cases both reflected, and contributed to, a major re-examination of adults' responsibility in ensuring that children's medical needs were met and prompted reconsiderations of the role of the state in enforcing that duty. As this history also demonstrates, however, a truly progressive vision of medical care as a right belonging to all children was neither universally shared nor long sustained.[8]

Chapter 2, The Physical Child, traces changing conceptualizations of children in scientific medicine over the course of the nineteenth century and the widespread dissemination of these ideas in popular domestic advice literature aimed at parents, particularly mothers. Physicians urged parents to scrutinize their children's bodies closely looking for signs and symptoms of possible danger and advised them about when, exactly, their children's care required the professional services of practitioners trained in scientific medicine. The emergence of pediatrics as a medical specialty secured a central place for physicians as experts in child-rearing. Chapter 3, The Public Child, examines the role of child welfare advocates in rendering children's physical well-being into matters requiring urgent societal attention. While early in the century reformers framed child welfare in terms of moral order and social stability, by century's end a new generation of advocates focused on the imperative of meeting children's physical needs and redefining child abuse and neglect in medicalized terms. Chapter 4, The Metaphysical Child, explores the healing paradigm that Mary Baker Eddy first laid out in her 1875 text, *Science and Health with Key to the Scriptures*, the foundation of the healing system that was central to the church she founded four years later in Lynn, Massachusetts. Eddy's denial of the reality of human sickness and her views concerning the immateriality of children's bodies stood in sharp contrast with contemporary trends that placed unprecedented importance on children's physical care, a disjuncture that soon led to conflicts between practitioners of spiritual and scientific healing and raised profound dilemmas for parents of sick and injured children.

Chapter 5, The Infected Child, highlights the pivotal role played by bacteriology in revolutionizing the theory and practice of scientific medicine, including the new field of pediatrics. Children were often regarded as the special beneficiaries of the new laboratory sciences, a promise that resonated with particular force after 1892 when diphtheria antitoxin came into use in the United States. Early enthusiasm for antitoxin's production and use, however, led to further conflict as public health leaders allied with physicians in private practice clashed with parents who rejected medical treatments for their children as a commitment to their religious faith. Chapter 6 focuses on the divine healer John Alexander Dowie whose noisy crusade against medical science in Chicago embroiled him in a series of clashes with local health authorities that brought attention to his movement far beyond that city. His followers faced both criminal charges and public opprobrium when they refused to seek medical care for family members, including infants and children. Chapter 7 traces the evolution of religious-based medical neglect in the courts, beginning in 1901 when an adherent of Dowie in Westchester County, New York became the first parent in the United States to be successfully prosecuted for manslaughter following the death of his daughter from bronchial pneumonia. The mixed outcomes of early twentieth-century criminal trials reflected Americans' ambivalence about the unwelcome incursion of the state into parental authority and prompted a backlash from those who insisted that such decisions constituted matters of personal and religious liberty.

Chapter 8 follows the narrative through the remainder of the twentieth century as the ascendancy of scientific medical practices, including successful campaigns to eradicate deadly childhood diseases such as diphtheria and polio, weakened a long-standing claim that spiritual and scientific healing represented equivalent treatments and therefore parents who relied on the former exclusively could not be held criminally responsible when their children died. Supporters of the rights of parents to reject scientific medicine therefore relied more heavily on the inclusion of special exemptions for religious healing within states' child abuse and neglect laws. In 1879, in *Reynolds v. U. S.*, the Supreme Court had delineated a line between belief and practice in determining the scope of constitutional protections for religious liberty. By the mid-twentieth century, however, the court had begun to broaden that scope, blurring the previous distinction between belief and practice and affording more protections for parents' religion-based choices in raising their children. After World War II pediatricians solidified their authority as experts in child-rearing, but they did so largely as private practitioners working in the absence of a broader movement dedicated to the proposition that children's health care represented a matter of shared national interest. Although medical advances continued to improve children's life chances and offered demonstrable means to assuage their physical suffering, fundamental questions about whether all children enjoy a right to benefit from the science of the age remained unresolved at the end of the twentieth century, and indeed lingered well into the twenty-first.

## Notes

1. Alexandra Minna Stern and Howard Markel, editors, *Formative Years: Children's Health in the United States, 1880–2000* (Ann Arbor: University of Michigan Press, 2004), 1–20; Evelynn Maxine Hammonds, *Childhood's*

*Deadly Scourge: The Campaign to Control Diphtheria in New York City, 1880–1930* (Baltimore: Johns Hopkins University Press, 1999), 10–11.

2. David S. Tanenhaus, "Between Dependency and Liberty: The Conundrum of Children's Rights in the Gilded Age," *Law and History Review*, Volume 23, Number 2 (Summer 2005): 351–385; Barbara Bennett Woodhouse, *Hidden in Plain Sight: The Tragedy of Children's Rights from Ben Franklin to Lionel Tate* (Princeton: Princeton University Press, 2008), 6–7.

3. Mark Douglas MacGarvie, *Law and Religion in American History: Public Values and Private Conscience* (New York: Cambridge University Press, 2016), 111–118; Stephen Gottschalk, *Rolling Away the Stone: Mary Baker Eddy's Challenge to Materialism* (Bloomington: Indiana University Press, 2006), 1–12. On Americans wrestling with science and modernity at the turn of the twentieth century, see T. J. Jackson Lears, *No Place of Grace: Antimodernism and the Transformation of American Culture, 1880–1920* (Pantheon Books, 1981).

4. Amanda Porterfield, *Healing in the History of Christianity* (New York: Oxford University Press, 2005), 3; Ronald L. Numbers, *Prophetess of Health: A Study of Ellen G. White*. Third edition (Grand Rapids, MI: Wm. B. Eerdmans Publishing Company, 2008), 239–266; Brian C. Wilson, *Dr. John Harvey Kellogg and the Religion of Biologic Living* (Bloomington: Indiana University Press, 2014), 30–61; Heather D. Curtis, *Faith in the Great Physician: Suffering and Divine Healing in American Culture, 1860–1900* (Baltimore: Johns Hopkins University Press, 2007), 156–157.

5. Michael C. Willrich, *Pox: An American History* (New York: Penguin, 2011).

6. "Religious Exemptions to Medical Care of Sick Children (As of 2017)." CHILD USA; Paul A. Offit, *Bad Faith: When Religious Belief Undermines Modern Medicine* (New York: Basic Books, 2015).

7. Martha Albertson Fineman, "What Is Right for Children?" In Martha Albertson Fineman and Karen Worthington, editors, *What Is Right for Children? The Competing Paradigms of Religion and Human Rights* (Burlington, VT: Ashgate, 2009), 1–6; Barbara Bennett Woodhouse, *Hidden in Plain Sight: The Tragedy of Children's Rights from Ben Franklin to Lionel Tate* (Princeton, NJ: Princeton University Press, 2008); Rennie B. Schoepflin, *Christian Science on Trial: Religious Healing on Trial* (Baltimore: Johns Hopkins University Press, 2003); Shawn Francis Peters, *When Prayer Fails: Faith Healing, Children, and the Law* (New York: Oxford University Press, 2008); Alan Rogers, *The Child Cases: How America's Religious Exemption Laws Harm Children* (Amherst: University of Massachusetts Press, 2014).

8. Vivian A. Zelizer, *Pricing the Priceless Child: The Changing Social Value of Children* (Princeton, NJ: Princeton University Press, 1985); Linda Gordon, "The Perils of Innocence, or What's Wrong with Putting Children First," *Journal of the History of Children and Youth*, Volume 1, Number 3 (Fall 2008): 332–350.

# CHAPTER 2

# The Physical Child

Who indeed does not perceive… that the maladies of infants and children form a class, in some measure apart from those of the adult; that they have their peculiar language; run often a very different course; and require for their cure a particular mode of treatment?

In 1844, the prominent Philadelphia physician David Francis Condie published the first edition of his influential work, *A Practical Treatise on the Diseases of Children*. In the text's introduction Condie stated his intention to provide "a simple statement of pathological facts, and plain therapeutic directions"—information that would relay to his readers his own professional "observations and experience acquired during a long and somewhat extensive practice." Although writing for an audience of American physicians, Condie consciously avoided abstract discourses on esoteric medical theories. Instead, he promoted the practice of directly observing children's physical states, offered recommendations for the daily feeding and hygiene of infants, and described pragmatic modes of treating childhood ailments. Condie's learned medical treatise therefore exhibited features more closely associated with the popular domestic advice manuals that proliferated in his time, contributing to what historian Carolyn Steedman has called a "veritable explosion of information" concerning the physiological development of children, their unique diseases, and their specific therapeutic needs. Since

L. Curry, *Religion, Law, and the Medical Neglect of Children in the United States, 1870–2000*, Palgrave Studies in the History of Childhood, https://doi.org/10.1007/978-3-030-24689-1_2

the late eighteenth century, an understanding had been steadily emerging that acknowledged childhood as a distinct phase in human growth, one that established critical foundations for the future adult's physical health and moral character. Further, as historian Crista DeLuzio has noted, a broader "discourse of development" found in novels, pedagogical treatises, and religious tracts extended the discussion far beyond the pages of medical books, disseminating concerns about the distinct phase of life known as childhood throughout American society. During the nineteenth century, the state of children's health took an unprecedented importance, both inside and outside of the walls of the private household.[1]

When it appeared in the 1840s, Condie's medical treatise stood atop a solid foundation of preceding texts written by doctors with the intention of relaying scientific information about children's physical states to a broad audience. In 1748, the British physician William Cadogan offered his *Essay Upon Nursing and the Management of Children, from Their Birth to Three Years of Age* as a corrective to what he perceived to be harmful mismanagement by lay nurses tasked with caring for foundling infants in London's institutions. In 1772, the Scottish physician William Buchan followed Cadogan's lead, producing the influential *Domestic Medicine, or, A Treatise on the Prevention and Cure of Diseases by Regimen and Simple Medicines*, much of which focused on the needs of children, including daily hygiene, diet, and exercise as well as treatment of childhood-specific diseases. Like many of his Enlightenment contemporaries, Buchan believed that lifelong predispositions to both disease and character weakness were formed in infancy; he therefore considered it essential that "parents be well acquainted with the various causes that may injure the health of their offspring." (Buchan had continental counterparts in the Swiss physician S. A. Tissot and the German Bernhard Christoph Faust.) Across the Atlantic, the many subsequent editions of Buchan's original treatise found their way to publishers in cities such as Baltimore, Boston, Hartford, Newark, and New York, reaching an American population that by 1790 approached four million people, half of whom were under sixteen years old. Thirty-five years later, Philadelphia obstetrician William Potts Dewees extended the scope of medical advice to include the prenatal period in *A Treatise on the Physical and Medical Treatment of Children*. "We have attempted to determine the influence of physical agents upon the constitution of the being," he explained in the manual's preface, "from its embryo existence to that state of development called puberty." Dewees wrote his treatise for an audience of practitioners who, even if formally trained, had little or no familiarity with the latest thinking about children's health care. Before the last half of the nineteenth century, medical training in the United States consisted primarily of attending lecture courses and serving an apprenticeship; reading texts therefore represented an important element of a physician's ongoing education. Dewees's treatise included a glossary explaining medical terms, arranged in alphabetical order from "abscess" to "weal." By the mid-nineteenth century literature addressing children's health had become a distinct mass market genre in the United States, uniting both physicians and lay readers in the belief that children required specialized, and scientifically managed, physical care.[2]

The male physicians who attempted to supplant traditional folk wisdom with the latest scientific medical advice on children's health care sought to justify the expansion of their professional purview into cultural spaces traditionally dominated by mothers, midwives, and nurses. "It is with great pleasure," Cadogan wrote in 1748, "I see at last the Preservation of Children Become the Care of Men of Sense." Buchan strongly advised against swaddling, a common midwifery custom in England and colonial America in which newborns were tightly wrapped in lengths of bandages supported with stiff stays. Such tightly bundled bodies rendered newborns easier to handle and arguably safer when they were placed in cradles and baskets. Buchan, however, believed that swaddling unnecessarily constrained and over-heated infants' bodies, risking deleterious effects on their health that might last a lifetime. His view echoed that of the Enlightenment philosopher and medical doctor John Locke who, in his 1693 essay *Some Thoughts Concerning Education*, had similarly proscribed against overheating. Very young children, Locke counseled, should be kept "not too warm and [in] straight clothing; especially the head and feet kept cold," a regimen he believed to be essential for strengthening children's moral as well as their physical constitutions. By 1825, the American physician William Dewees heralded the triumph of the medical crusade against swaddling, referring to the largely discarded "cruel and absurd" practice as the relic of a benighted past. In the United States, physicians only grew more assertive in the second half of the nineteenth century, particularly after 1880 when the field of pediatrics emerged as a separate and distinct medical specialization.[3]

But, rather than entirely supplanting traditional domestic roles, elevating the importance of children's bodies required the formation of a partnership between formally trained "regular" doctors and parents, particularly mothers who were best positioned to make close daily observations of their children's physical states and to report signs of trouble to physicians. While nineteenth-century doctors battled what they deemed to be outmoded folk practices, they just as consistently blamed parental *indifference* as a threat to children's well-being. "Loss of time is often the greatest possible consequence," Dewees warned in 1825, "since it permits a disease of a dangerous character to take an insidious, or too often a fatal hold, before the danger is suspected, or the proper remedy applied." Constant vigilance over the child's body was required, and therefore the careless, distracted, or overworked parent was as much to be lamented as the uninformed one. While doctors directed most of their scolding at mothers, establishing what historian Kathleen M. Brown has called "new health and class-driven imperatives to provide scrupulous and intimate care for children's bodies," men did not entirely escape censure for neglecting parental responsibilities. Dewees warned that the demanding task of constantly monitoring a child's health inevitably led to the overtaxing of its mother. He advised that relieving the maternal burden "can most profitably be done by the father partaking in this arduous and interesting duty." Well aware that his counsel might cause a stir in some households, the physician ruefully acknowledged that modifying gender expectations would be difficult because "unfortunately at present everything connected to the nursery and education is voted a bore by the modern fine gentleman, and the physical treatment of his children is a duty he would feel almost disgraced to perform." For Dewees and his medical contemporaries, the enlightened and scientific care of children deserved the serious attention of men as well as women, of inexpert parents as well as educated physicians.[4]

It is difficult to know precisely how lay audiences understood, evaluated, and applied the information proffered in the pages of domestic medical manuals. Historian Karin Calvert has argued that in the early 1800s marked changes in the material culture of the household suggest that many parents were indeed abandoning traditional child-rearing customs and aligning domestic practices more closely to Enlightenment precepts. The sheer abundance of titles on the market by the middle of the century demonstrates the emergence of a sizable, literate, and likely middle-class readership that regarded the scientifically based medical care of children to be a subject worthy of their interest, even if time and resources limited their ability to apply what they read within their parenting practices. In transmitting the latest views on infant and child health care from important centers of western medical education such as Edinburgh and Philadelphia, physicians assumed their lay readers, both male and female, could follow instructions couched in scientific, or quasi-scientific, language. William

Buchan's elaborate subtitle, "being an attempt to render the medical art more generally useful, by shewing people what is in their own power both with respect to the prevention and cure of diseases," clearly signaled his intention to educate parents in the scientific medical management of their households. The many subsequent editions of Buchan's treatise continued to find a receptive American audience for several decades.[5]

Buchan's work followed two extremely popular predecessors in England and America, the anonymously authored *Every Man His Own Doctor* published by Benjamin Franklin in 1737 and *Primitive Physick*, written by the clergyman John Wesley in 1747. These works, however, had been authored by nonphysicians and had promoted self-diagnosis and the virtue of trusting one's own experience over taking direction from formally trained medical men— untrustworthy sorts who often shrouded their healing practices in arcane theories and proprietary dogma. The tract published by Franklin was expressly advertised as a work "design'd for those who can't afford to dye by the Hand of a Doctor." In contrast to *Every Man*'s anti-intellectualism, Buchan's *Domestic Medicine* advanced the notion that obtaining scientific medical knowledge empowered lay people to take effective measures in preventing and even curing the diseases that afflicted their household members. In 1807, James Ewell promoted his manual entitled *The Medical Companion, or Family Physician*, as a work aimed at a distinctly American readership, to be read by both medical students and laypersons who "live in the country, or who go to sea, where regular and timely assistance cannot always be obtained." Historians recognize an 1811 work, *The Maternal Physician: A Treatise on the Nurture and Management of Infants, from Birth Until Two Years Old. Being the Result of Sixteen Years' Experience in the Nursery*, as the first American manual that addressed the subject of children's health specifically. Authored by "An American Matron," later identified as a Philadelphia woman named Mary Palmer Tyler, the text was in large part a compendium of information gleaned from contemporary medical treatises intermingled with Tyler's own experiences in child-rearing. The broad reach of this literature carved out a distinctive role for parents and doctors to act in consort in applying the latest scientific precepts to children's health care. In so doing, it also advanced and legitimized the physical care of children as a subject worthy of attention in the education and training of regular medical practitioners.[6]

Until the mid-nineteenth century, doctors and their adult patients shared a basic underlying frame of reference for matters concerning health and disease. Optimal health required incessant monitoring and adjusting of daily "intake and outflow" as bodily systems continuously interacted with the surrounding environment. This view reflected an ancient western medical paradigm, originating with Aristotle and developed in the third century by the Roman physician Galen, premised on the existence of four "humors" (*chymoi*)—universal elements whose qualities took organic form within the human body. Made up of intangible matter rather than observable substances, the humors functioned as explanatory metaphors for understanding an individual's bodily state at any given point in time. Because an imbalance of humors caused physical illness as well as faulty personal temperament, the goal was to maintain moderation in both bodily habits and personal passions. The key to optimal health lay in maintaining equilibrium, and therefore physicians and patients alike paid close attention to the body's near-constant natural fluctuations. Doctors might employ "physic" to restore the balanced state—dosing patients with quinine to alleviate fevers, for example—but never without prescribing an accompanying regimen of diet, exercise, and rest aimed at maintaining humoral stability. While over time numerous innovations modified Galen's original paradigm, its basic framework remained intact for nearly fifteen centuries. Historian Richard A. Meckel has noted that the explanatory power of the equilibrium metaphor served to unite the otherwise diverse health care universe of the early nineteenth century. The drastic nature of "heroic" therapeutic interventions such as bloodletting, sweating, and purging employed by regular doctors produced a strong protest reaction in the form of alternative healing sects such as homeopathy, hydropathy, and Thomsonianism—alternative schools of healing that attracted considerable followings in the antebellum United States. But, whether they dosed their patients with botanicals, water, or other material medica, practitioners of both regular and sectarian medicine intervened in bodily systems with the objective of correcting an unbalanced state, a goal that required communication and active collaboration with the patient.[7]

Children's continual physical development provoked frequent periods of disequilibrium, making caring for their health an especially urgent case for cooperation between physicians and parents. A long-held view shared by physicians and nonphysicians alike regarded young children as "choleric," or naturally disposed to an overabundance of choler, a humor produced by the liver and resting in the bowels. Also known as red and yellow bile, in the humoral model choler was associated with the element of fire and believed to stir heat and agitation within the body. Medieval European physicians theorized that skin eruptions, including smallpox and measles, occurred in young children because their blood had been kept extremely warm in utero, reaching a near-boiling point during the strenuous birthing process. They warned that common cultural practices such as feeding babies diets only appropriate for adults, including stimulating alcoholic drinks, only served to exacerbate their naturally over-excited constitutions. Curing scrofula (clusters of hard nodes that ulcerated the skin), required "treating all things that fill the head with fumes," from garlic and strong wine to "shouting, worry, and anger." While of course medical views evolved over the centuries, concerns about babies' natural tendency to overproduce bile long remained an underlying tenet of both scientific and folk medicine. In the late eighteenth century, William Buchan decried a long-held custom of treating scrofula with strong purgatives in order to rid children's bodies of "gross choler," noting that such harsh nostrums used by parents and physicians alike debilitated little ones' systems and further aggravated disease. (Buchan preferred the remedy of bathing scrofulous children in salt water as a means of correcting the unbalanced state.) But, if the Scottish physician rejected the purging of bile by drastic means, he nevertheless retained the view that the source of very young children's ailments lays in their bowels, the site where choler resided. In a distressing feedback loop, babies' choleric make-up predisposed them to general states of nervous agitation, or colic, stimulating the production of bile, which in turn caused a range of gastro-intestinal complaints. Left untreated, colicky babies were at risk for debilitated bodies as well as flawed characters.[8]

In his 1825 treatise the American physician William Dewees differentiated between two types of colic. The first consisted of acute periods of gastric distress occurring at various points throughout the day. Dewees attributed these attacks to several dietary causes, including inappropriate foods, over-feeding, and mother's milk that was "ill-elaborated," or lacking in vital power. To remedy the latter he advised nursing mothers to undertake a complete change of their own dietary habits, accompanied by a regimen of "well-regulated exercise." In the meantime, while mothers brought their own bodily systems into proper balance, more immediate measures for relieving the child's gastric distress included administering minute doses of magnesia (magnesium oxide) and warm sweet oil. A second form of colic made its appearance at the same time each day regardless of the dietary circumstances of mother or baby. Dewees attributed this condition to the individual "constitutional peculiarity" of the child itself. Assuring parents that this type of colic was concerning but never dangerous, the physician promised it would naturally "wear itself out" in two or three months. Writing twenty years later, David Francis Condie was considerably less sanguine about the risks associated with babies' colicky constitutions. "During the entire period of infancy the nervous susceptibility is particularly acute," he asserted, "all impressions are vividly felt, though usually transient in their effects. Sympathetic affections from reflex actions are readily induced, and often give rise to irregular or morbid action from trifling irritations." Condie maintained that, if left unmitigated, a baby's naturally nervous temperament could be made manifest in the form of bodily fevers and convulsions. Listed under the heading "gastro-enteric irritations," his treatise addressed external, observable manifestations of the inner choleretic state such as eczema, herpes, psoriasis, tumors, and warts.[9]

Hippocrates had regarded teething as one of the most destabilizing and dangerous periods in children's development, and concern for dentition's acute hazards remained apparent in western medical practice and cultural custom well into the nineteenth century. In 1789, William Buchan attributed fully one-tenth of all infant deaths in Great Britain to complications of the dentition process. Nevertheless, the physician recommended against a common medical practice of his time in which the physician lanced an infant's gums to aid the erupting tooth. Interestingly, the "maternal physician" Mary Palmer Tyler urged her readers to learn to perform the procedure themselves, advising them to "to cut [the gums] with a very keen razor while the infant sleeps." Less adventuresome mothers could choose from among a range of material objects specially designed to see babies safely through the ordeal of teething. In 1833 John Eberle, a founder of the Jefferson Medical College in Philadelphia, devoted nineteen pages to the subject of dentition in his text, *A Treatise on the Diseases and Physical Education of Children*. Eberle described teething as a "deviation from the healthy condition of the system" in which the infant "manifests an irritable and fretful temper" and even "slight exciting causes are apt to give rise to febrile irritation." While Eberle did not believe dentition itself to be significant as a direct cause of infant death, he did assert that the compromised bodily state it engendered allowed other diseases to "acquire a fatal violence" if they were contracted during the teething period. Such dire forebodings understandably caused attentive parents a great deal of worry, as evidenced by the anxieties expressed by middle-class mothers in their correspondence and journals. In 1825, for example, new mother Elizabeth Ellery Sedgwick confessed in her diary that she was "filled with terror" at the prospect of her baby's future teething. Sedgwick's private maternal concerns were shared by the medical community existing well beyond her New York household. The *American Journal of Medical Sciences*, which began publishing in Philadelphia in 1820, identified teething among causes of death in its reported mortality statistics. Fifty years later, the Chicago Board of Health listed dentition as one of that Midwestern city's leading causes of infant death.[10]

If such anxieties forged a common bond of concern between parents and physicians, both parties absolutely dreaded the arrival of a particularly virulent range diarrheal diseases known colloquially as "summer complaint." As its vernacular name suggests, this form of gastro-intestinal malady was widely observed to run rampant during periods of hot weather. It could appear very suddenly in seemingly healthy children, causing intense suffering, and provoked a rapid wasting in its victims that all too often proved fatal, killing perhaps tens of thousands of babies and young children annually in the United States. Its widespread prevalence, as well as its acute deadliness, rendered summer complaint a topic of utmost concern among the American medical community. It caught the attention of the prominent Philadelphia physician Benjamin Rush who in 1777 published *An Inquiry into the Causes and Cure of the Cholera Infantum*, the first medical treatise to formally name and address this most feared and mysterious disease. As a practitioner of internal medicine Rush treated large numbers of children and spent considerable time observing and treating their bodily states. He also took an academic interest in children's special needs for medical care, addressing various related topics in lectures and scholarly articles.[11]

Rush theorized that, because babies lacked teeth, their bodies produced an excess of gastric juices designed to aid in the digestion of food. This natural excess could be further excited by external stimuli such as light, sound, heat, and air, with potentially harmful consequences to a child's health. Like most of his medical contemporaries, Rush believed that cholera infantum occurred more frequently in towns than in rural areas and was more widespread in America than in Europe. He attributed its higher incidence to the peculiarities of the American diet and the generally warmer climate of the United States. The most significant factor, however, was the lack of fresh air endemic to summer months in cities such as his own Philadelphia, a notoriously unhealthy locale where "at each inhaling of air, one worries about the next." As prophylaxis Rush counseled daily cold baths for children, dressing them in seasonally appropriate clothing, offering them periodic sips of diluted wine and, if at all possible, relocating them from the city to the country during long stretches of hot weather. Such measures assumed both that parents would be adequately informed about measures to prevent cholera infantum and that they possessed sufficient means to carry them out. Rush also promoted a key role for physicians once the dreaded disease had been contracted. An ardent advocate of bloodletting to relieve fevers and other "inflammatory states," he was considerably less conservative than were his contemporaries in using that drastic remedy to treat children, even very young ones. In 1796 Rush published a treatise entitled *Defense of Bloodletting* in response to growing professional opposition to the practice. He argued that, despite posing health risks of its own, the timely use of bloodletting had more often than not "snatched children from the grave." Always one to practice what he preached, the doctor bled his own infant son and daughter when they suffered from fevers at just a few weeks of age. Happily, both infants survived their ordeals.[12]

Nearly fifty years after the publication of Rush's study another Philadelphia physician, William Potts Dewees, devoted twelve pages of his own treatise to the causes, symptoms, and treatment of cholera infantum. Significantly, Dewees provided a vivid and detailed account of the outward manifestations that distinguished the serious disease from common colic and other more benign gastro-intestinal complaints. He described a set of readily observable symptoms that could alert informed and attentive parents to the true danger of their child's condition. "We have few diseases in which the emaciation of the patient so rapidly takes place," the physician noted, "or where, in its later stages, there is a greater alteration of general condition and aspect." From this unusually rapid onset, an equally precipitous decline followed, which Dewees further elucidated in disturbing detail:

> The child at first becomes pallid, and the flesh flabby; and so completely is the fat ultimately absorbed, that the integuments [skin] hang in folds; and in those parts on which the body rests, livid spots appear, followed by ulcerations. The skin on the forehead is tight, as if bound to the bone; the eyes are sunk; the cheeks fall in; the nose is sharp; and the lips are shrivelled [sic].[13]

Dewees went on to cite several simple treatments parents could attempt on their own, such as giving the child teaspoons of warm salt water or black coffee to drink, interventions he believed would calm overexcited stomach and bowels. He also suggested parents administer minute doses of calomel (mercurous oxide), a purgative substance that was widely used to treat children's ailments despite being both harsh and dangerous. Should these first-tier remedies prove ineffective and the child's symptoms worsen, Dewees advised more technical measures that required the skilled services of a physician, including bleeding, blistering, and the administration of complex compound substances, for which he provided exact mixing and dosing instructions. Dewees's frightening description of cholera infantum's wasting symptoms provided more than a tutorial on the disease for medical practitioners. His unsparing prose also sent a clear warning that children's bodily states must be observed closely and constantly, with attending adults remaining ever alert to changes indicating potential peril. In cases of cholera infantum, as Dewees's graphic illustration made clear, inattentiveness to a child's rapidly deteriorating condition could have tragic consequences. It was therefore imperative that parents recognize when their own efforts were inadequate and the time had come to seek out the expert interventions of a trained physician.[14]

Dewees's stress on the importance of close observation was magnified twenty years later when David Francis Condie asserted that minute inspections of children's bodies formed the "principle source of diagnosis" in detecting their underlying ailments. "As a preliminary to the study of the semeiology [sic] of the disease of infancy," he wrote in *A Practical Treatise on the Diseases of Children*, "it is essential that the physician should make himself fully acquainted with the external appearance of the infant during health." Advanced scientific medicine therefore required doctors to pay very close attention to the unique attributes of children's bodies—how they appeared to the outside observer in both sickness and in health. In an elaborate description sustained over twenty pages of text, Condie outlined a technique in which the physician carefully and holistically scrutinized a young patient, noting "the expressions of the countenance—the gestures—the phenomena of sleep—the mode in which respiration is effected—the cry—the condition of the tongue and mouth—the condition of the surface—the state of the breath—the evacuations." It was incumbent upon the doctor to retain a detailed record of such observations in order to better identify any potentially dangerous alterations that might occur in the child's bodily systems. "Our attention will probably be first attracted by some underlying *change*," he emphasized, "which it will require a stricter observation to decypher [sic], and associate with its peculiar cause." The "medical gaze" that Condie advocated reflected an underlying historical process in which western medicine was moving away from the ancient humoral paradigm rooted in metaphor and speculation and toward an empirical science based on observation and identification. Appearing in 1844, Condie's detailed instructions for the physical examination of children assumed the uniqueness of the child's body in comparison to that of the adult and, what is more, promoted the notion that children's bodily states in both sickness and health had a place in medical science.[15]

In the first half of the nineteenth century, American medical writing on children consisted of "a curious array in which symptoms, diseases, hygienic matters, comments on psychology, and the meconium were thrown together in what appeared to be a purely arbitrary manner," according to historian Thomas E. Cone. The ability to actually cure diseases once they had been contracted remained as formidable a challenge to David Francis Condie as it had to Benjamin Rush; proportionate to all deaths, as many children under five years of age died in 1850 as in 1789. Unlike its European counterparts, particularly in France and Germany where university-based education was the pre-eminent means of training doctors, American medicine had not strongly emphasized laboratory and clinical medicine. Physicians in the United States awarded a greater value to learning from their colleagues' personal experiences in attending patients at the bedside, a product of a long tradition in which young doctors had been trained through years of apprenticeship. What is more, the fading but still evident influence of the humoral paradigm kept medical care focused on the individual patient's "intake and outflow"—restoring and maintaining a balanced bodily state—rather than identifying and addressing diseases as specific entities. By mid-century, however, a complete reorientation in children's medical care, one that aligned American physicians more closely with their French and German counterparts, lay just on the horizon.[16]

In 1848, John Forsyth Meigs published an influential text entitled *A Practical Treatise on the Diseases of Children*. A physician and lecturer on children's diseases at the Philadelphia Medical Association, Meigs was highly critical of the merely "anecdotal" nature of most medical literature in the United States. Unlike many earlier works, Meigs's own treatise was logically organized according to specific diseases that affected particular bodily systems, including pneumonia, hooping [sic] cough, scarlet fever, and measles. (True to American tradition, Meigs did occasionally depart from his categorical discussions to offer illustrative anecdotes from his own professional experience.) The following year the physician John R. Beck published *Essays on Infant Therapeutics* in which he considered the particularized effects of a series of common allopathic remedies on children's unique bodily systems including opium, mercury, ergot, emetics, and bloodletting. He noted, for example, that opium acted both with greater "energy" and with greater "uncertainty" in young patients than in adults. Beck counseled doctors to consider a range of individual variables such as the child's sex and race, as well as environmental factors like season and temperature, in determining appropriate dosages. As the publications by Meigs and Beck demonstrate, after the midpoint of the nineteenth century the scientific literature on children's medical care had begun to diverge from the genre of popular domestic advice manuals with which it had shared a common heritage. As the contours of a new medical specialty took shape, physicians trained in clinical and laboratory sciences began to play a larger role as experts in understanding and addressing the diseases of childhood.[17]

In 1860 Abraham Jacobi arrived at the New York Medical College, marking a watershed in the evolution of American pediatric medicine. Jacobi graduated from Bonn University in Germany, where his training had been centered on the laboratory sciences. Between 1850 and 1880 the institution of the laboratory transformed German medical education, as evidenced by the emergence of new and specialized fields of study including anatomy, physiology, and pathology. While at Bonn University, however, Jacobi did not limit his interests to his medical studies. He became caught up in the revolutionary politics of 1848, and in fact served two successive prison sentences as a result of his radical activism. In 1853 Jacobi followed Karl Marx and Friedrich Engels in seeking political asylum in England, where he tried, unsuccessfully, to establish himself as a physician. After several months of frustration, Jacobi decided to leave England and try his luck practicing medicine in the United States.[18]

Jacobi's first American medical experience was as a physician serving the poor German immigrant community in New York City's Lower East Side, a district whose exceptionally high rate of infant mortality could hardly have escaped his attention. Along with several like-minded colleagues Jacobi founded the German Dispensary of New York, modeled on the German university clinics with which he was familiar. The new facility offered free medical services to poor families. Jacobi and his colleagues treated over seventeen hundred children in its first year of operation; twenty-five years later, Jacobi estimated that German Dispensary physicians had attended some 350,000 cases. In time the physician drew upon this extensive clinical experience to write a series of essays on the pathology and therapeutics of infancy, a contribution to the medical literature that, according to historian

Russell Viner, "revolutionized the way Americans understood the diseases of children." Subsequently, the second half of the nineteenth century saw a proliferation of clinics, dispensaries, and hospitals that addressed the health care of children exclusively, most of them from poor and working-class families. Within two the span of two decades clinics and hospitals specializing in treating childhood diseases were established in New York, Boston, Washington, Philadelphia, San Francisco, Chicago, St. Louis, and Cincinnati. While historically health care institutions had served the purpose of isolating (as opposed to curing) the sick, they now emerged as critical sites for the education and training of physicians. These institutions provided doctors with a solid foundation of clinical observation that soon propelled pediatrics into a full-fledged medical specialty, a separate field distinct from both adult and obstetrical medicine. Attesting to pediatrics' rapid growth and expanding influence, the period between 1850 and 1900 saw a ten-fold increase in scientific publications addressing the diseases of childhood.[19]

With three years' experience at the German Dispensary under his belt, Abraham Jacobi arrived at the New York Medical College having been granted the title "professor of infantile pathology and therapeutics," a position from which he delivered weekly lectures to doctors interested in pursuing the new specialty. In 1873 Jacobi married the physician Mary Putnam, who served on the faculty of the Woman's Medical College of the New York Infirmary where in 1886 she established a dedicated children's ward. A graduate of the École de Médicine in Paris, Putnam Jacobi was an influential figure in her own right, having gained recognition for promoting the integration of clinical and laboratory medicine in the United States. Like Abraham and Mary Putnam Jacobi, Job Lewis Smith's career illustrates a common trajectory among the first generation of American pediatricians, from the clinic and dispensary to the university. Smith, an 1853 graduate of the New York College of Physicians and Surgeons, established a practice in far uptown Manhattan where he encountered a population doing its best to survive in poorly constructed tenements built on streets sorely lacking in sewers and drains. Not surprisingly, the neighborhood was plagued by high rates of infant and childhood mortality, with diarrheal diseases as a significant cause. Smith's experience practicing among the local residents eventually propelled him to a post as professor of children's diseases and pathology at Bellevue Hospital.[20] In 1869 he published what would become an extremely influential medical textbook based largely on his own clinical experience as well as his expertise in the laboratory. *A Treatise on the Diseases of Infancy and Childhood* would be revised and reissued eight times over the next thirty years. In the text's introduction Smith stated the case for pediatrics as its own medical specialty in candid terms:

> Diseases in early life differ in important particulars from those occurring in maturity. Some which are common in the former age are unknown in the latter, and those which occur equally at all ages often present peculiar symptoms and a peculiar clinical history in the young. Therefore physicians who are skilled in treating adults, may be unskillful in treating children. Excellence as a physician of children can only be achieved by special and continued study of their ailments.[21]

Smith's lengthy and detailed descriptions (the text ran to well over seven hundred pages) systematically addressed a long list of illnesses specific to, or else commonly occurring in, childhood including infantile paralysis, cholera infantum, and diphtheria. Beginning with the prenatal period, Smith arranged the book categorically according to the bodily systems affected, ending with an appendix that covered the topic of infant feeding, a feature that notably included his own assessments of a number of commercially available products that he listed by name.

Unlike his forebears earlier in the century, demystifying children's health care for a broad readership clearly did not count among Smith's objectives. *A Treatise on the Diseases of Infancy and Childhood* was a medical text written exclusively for doctors. It employed highly technical language and assumed the reader had at least a foundational knowledge of scientific principles. Nevertheless, Smith's treatise reflected what historians have observed to be the peculiarly holistic nature of pediatrics in an age of increasing specialization in medical education and practice. Unlike other fields pediatrics grew, not from the discovery of a single organ or system, but rather from the recognition of childhood as a distinct stage in human development. From its earliest origins, therefore, pediatrics was both specialized and general in orientation, focusing on the uniqueness of the child's body while also encompassing a range of scientific disciplines such as anatomy, physiology, bacteriology, and pathology. Further, because pediatricians concerned themselves not only with bodily systems and functions but also with how children actually lived, the new specialty also freely crossed boundaries between scientific medicine and social reform. In the last decades of the nineteenth-century pediatricians cast a wide net in defining their professional purview, solidifying their formal organization in 1880 when the American Medical Association established a new division, the

Section on the Diseases of Children. Four years later, a dedicated medical journal, the *Archives of Pediatrics* began publication. These developmental milestones set the stage for the founding of the American Pediatric Society (APS) in 1888, with Abraham Jacobi serving as the organization's first president. The APS served a dual role in both advancing scientific understanding of children's physical care and promoting elite standards of education and training for doctors practicing the new specialty.[22]

At century's end American pediatrics had come into its own. In 1896 Luther Emmett Holt, a professor of the diseases of children at the New York Polyclinic, published what would become the most influential pediatric textbook to date, both inside and outside of the United States. (New editions of *The Diseases of Infancy and Childhood* were released into the 1940s.) In the text's introduction, Holt explained that the proceeding information resulted from his "eleven years' continuous service among young children" in clinical settings, a professional advantage that he hoped to make useful to "those whose opportunities for the study of disease in children are limited to the bedside." As promised, Holt's text considerably widened the horizons of physicians in private practice. It contained no fewer than one hundred and eighty-five illustrations, including artists' renderings showing the appearance of diseased organs and histograms that correlated higher rates of infant mortality with higher outdoor temperatures. Finally, there were schematic diagrams of several new technologies that formed an arsenal of modern weaponry newly available in the fight against infant and child mortality, including a laryngeal tube for inflating the lungs, a mechanical device for pasteurizing cow's milk, and an infant incubator for housing premature babies.[23]

A distinguishing feature of Holt's textbook was its emphasis on children's growth as a reflection of their overall health, an idea reinforced by the inclusion of charts that correlated ages with optimal heights and weights. Holt's discussion drew upon the work of Harvard University's Henry P. Bowditch who, beginning in the 1870s, had systematically studied the heights and weights of over twenty-five thousand schoolchildren in an attempt to identify factors that could explain individual variations. Bowditch's methodology followed the lead of mid-nineteenth-century actuaries who had begun constructing height and weight tables used by life insurance companies to determine adults' physical fitness. His research inspired a number of physicians to embark on a program of studying children's heights and weights in clinical settings, an effort that did produce notable statistical correlations among physical underdevelopment, the presence of disease, and increased rates of mortality. The next step was to construct standards for children's growth on the theory that significant deviations from the norm would alert doctors that a child's health was in some way compromised. Even more optimistically, pediatric researchers theorized that a program of weighing and measuring children might lead to effective interventions to prevent, or perhaps even cure, a number of childhood diseases. Holt's textbook drew upon these new standards and also widely promoted their use among practicing physicians. He recommended that babies be weighed weekly as a means of monitoring their health status. In the text's second edition, published in 1899, Holt justified giving extended coverage to the topic of weighing and measuring because its importance as a diagnostic tool was increasingly being recognized within the regular medical profession. For example rickets, a common but serious affliction with lifelong consequences for its victims, was not in fact a hereditary condition as once was commonly believed. What is more, because rickets resulted from poor nutrition, it was entirely preventable with adequate attention to a child's diet. Aided by Holt's influential textbook, the practice of systematically tracking height and weight soon became a standardized part of children's health care, not only in doctors' offices but anywhere that children were brought together in significant numbers including schools, orphan asylums, and settlement houses.[24]

After 1880, with its formal organization firmly established in the United States, pediatrics entered a new phase of accelerated growth and influence that continued unabated into the twentieth century. This era was also marked by vigorous efforts on the part of regular doctors, working through their own state-level organizations as well as the American Medical Association (founded in 1847 and incorporated fifty years later) to discredit and marginalize their sectarian competitors, most particularly practitioners of homeopathy. As states began setting higher standards for medical education and stricter credentials for medical licenses parents' own options in caring for their children's health became narrower. The phrase "practitioner of medicine" increasingly came to mean a regular physician who had been trained in an accredited institution and licensed by the state. By the early twentieth century regular medical doctors, especially those practicing the new field of pediatrics, had outdistanced their competitors in alternative healing sects, extending their professional reach in caring for children's health and broadening their social authority as overseers of children's well-being.[25]

As pediatrics coalesced into a distinct field within regular medicine—one that drew upon the latest discoveries in the laboratory sciences, built upon practitioners' extensive clinical experience, and endeavored to advance the understanding of children's health and the diseases of childhood—the gap between physicians and children's traditional caregivers grew wider. Previous generations had been united by a common understanding that health and disease were determined by the particular balance of humors existing within an individual's body. Thus they had not experienced a wide epistemological divide between medical science and lay healing. In the late eighteenth and early nineteenth centuries, the market for literature concerning children's physical care had encompassed all those concerned with the daily care of infants as well as any person who attended at the bedsides of sick children. By contrast, when Luther Emmett Holt's *The Diseases of Infancy and Childhood* appeared at century's end, it carried the subtitle *For the Use of Students and Practitioners of Medicine*, a clear indication that the text was intended for the edification of physicians who were formally trained and legally engaged in the practice of regular medicine.

If physicians increasingly encroached upon parents' traditional cultural space in caring for children's health, by no means did they seek to displace them at the bedside entirely. As their forebears had done, medical doctors of the late nineteenth century continued to depend heavily upon an active and cooperative partnership with parents. More than ever before, children's bodies required close and constant scrutiny to both determine their general state of health and to detect the possible presence of disease. Engaged in daily and intimate contact with their children parents, especially mothers, were the caregivers best situated to make crucial observations of bodily states, keep meticulous track of growth and weight gain, and understand when it was time to alert a physician to possible dangers. New standards for children's medical care brought about a revised set of social expectations about the nature and extent of parents' duties toward their children, obligations that now included seeking out the services of a physician—ideally a formally trained and licensed practitioner of regular medicine—when a child's well-being warranted that they do so. Under the new medical paradigm, parents did not need to understand the latest science that informed their children's health care. Rather, they needed to trust that *doctors* understood the latest science, and to accept a physician's professional judgment in place of their own parental prerogatives.

At the end of the nineteenth century, regular medicine promoted an acceptance of science most likely to be found among populations that were proficiently literate and enjoyed at least a middle-class standing. But bourgeois status did not automatically correlate with uncritical faith in the powers of regular medical practitioners. Certainly, the urban clinics and hospitals that played so vital a role in pediatrics' development as a medical field relied in no small measure on the willingness of poor and working-class families to cede the care of their little ones to doctors—including those to whom they were virtual strangers. At the same time, resistance to the state-supported hegemony that regular doctors increasingly enjoyed provoked a vigorous backlash from some middle-class citizens who protested measures such as exclusionary medical licensing and compulsory vaccination against smallpox. Just as significantly, during the last quarter of the century a number of new healing religions emerged whose doctrines entirely rejected the growing social and cultural dominance of science in American life. Despite being challenged by regular physicians, an array of secular and religious healing sects remained attractive to parents caring for sick and injured children. As long as all options enjoyed a roughly equal chance of success, parents' duties did not require them to choose one particular healing regime over another. But such broad parental freedoms to raise children exactly as they saw fit came under closer scrutiny at the turn of the twentieth century, when new medical practices rooted in the laboratory sciences offered for the first time demonstrably effective means for preventing, and even curing, some childhood diseases. A troubling question arose from this development: When new medical therapies became available, were parents legally obligated to seek them for their sick children?

From its initial appearance in the mid-nineteenth century, pediatrics claimed a broad scope for its professional interests and an equally expansive jurisdiction for its social authority. Building their specialty through observing, weighing, and measuring children's bodies within the confined spaces of households, clinics, and hospitals, pediatricians also looked outward, making common cause with public health and social reformers in crusades to reduce infant and childhood mortality. Since the late eighteenth century, an Enlightenment discourse of human development had stressed the importance of early childhood influences in producing future citizens who were both physically fit and morally sound. Over time, this generalized discourse coalesced into broad public action, producing a "child saving" movement predicated on the notion that children's well-being constituted a matter of public, not merely parental, concern. Campaigns against child labor, physical abuse, and parental neglect placed unprecedented significance on a societal duty to scrutinize, monitor, and protect children's bodies.

# NOTES

1. David Francis Condie, *A Practical Treatise on the Diseases of Children*. Second edition (Philadelphia: Lea and Blanchard, 1847), vii; Carolyn Steedman, *Strange Dislocations: Childhood and the Idea of Human Interiority, 1789–1830* (Cambridge: Harvard University Press, 1995), 5; Crista DeLuzio, *Female Adolescence in American Scientific Thought, 1830–1930* (Baltimore: Johns Hopkins University Press, 2007), 11–12.

2. William Cadogan, *An Essay Upon Nursing and the Management of Children from Their Birth to Three Years of Age* (London: Jay Roberts, 1748); William Buchan, *Domestic Medicine; or the Family Physician* (Philadelphia: John Dunlap, 1772 and Ann Arbor: Text Creation Partnership, 2008); William Potts Dewees, *A Treatise on the Physical and Medical Treatment of Children* (Philadelphia: H. C. Carey and I. Lea, 1825), xiv. On domestic medical manuals as a historical literary genre see Charles E. Rosenberg, "Health in the Home: A Tradition of Print and Practice," in Charles E. Rosenberg, editor, *Right Living: An Anglo-American Tradition of Self-Help Medicine and Hygiene* (Baltimore: Johns Hopkins University Press, 2003), 1–20; William H. Schmidt, "Health and Welfare of Colonial American Children," *American Journal of Diseases of Children*, Volume 130 (July 1976): 694–701; John Duffy, *From Humors to Medical Science: A History of American Medicine*. Second edition (Urbana: University of Illinois Press, 1993), 93; Richard A. Meckel, *Save the Babies: American Public Health Reform and the Prevention of Infant Mortality, 1850–1929* (Baltimore: Johns Hopkins University Press, 1990), 48–49.

3. Cadogan, *An Essay Upon Nursing and the Management of Children*, 3; Buchan, *Domestic Medicine*, 1; John Locke, *Some Thoughts Concerning Education* (London: Ward, Lock, and Company, 1693), 418. Historian Karin Calvert discusses the practice of swaddling newborns in colonial America in *Children in the House: The Material Culture of Early Childhood, 1600–1900* (Boston: Northeastern University Press, 1992), 19–26.

4. Dewees, *A Treatise on the Physical and Medical Treatment of Children*, vi, xiii; Kathleen M. Brown, *Foul Bodies: Cleanliness in Early America* (New Haven, CT: Yale University Press, 2007), 194.

5. Calvert, *Children in the House*, 56.

6. Stanley Finger, *Doctor Franklin's Medicine* (Philadelphia: University of Pennsylvania Press, 2006), 26; Duffy, *From Humors to Medical Science*, 93; Janet Golden, Richard A. Meckel, and Heather Munroe Prescott, editors, *Children and Youth in Sickness and in Health* (Westport, CT: Greenwood Press, 2004), 143.

7. John S. Haller Jr., *American Medicine in Transition 1840–1910* (Urbana: University of Illinois Press, 1981), 11; Roy Porter, *Flesh in the Age of Reason: The Modern Foundations of Body and Soul* (New York: W. W. Norton, 2003), 49–52; Charles E. Rosenberg, "The Therapeutic Revolution: Medicine, Meaning, and Social Change in Nineteenth-Century America."

In Morris J. Vogel and Charles E. Rosenberg, editors, *The Therapeutic Revolution: Essays in the Social History of American Medicine* (Philadelphia: University of Pennsylvania Press, 1979), 3–25; Luke Demaitre, *Medieval Medicine: The Art of Healing, from Head to Toe* (Santa Barbara: Praeger, 2013), 16; Meckel, *Save the Babies*, 22.

8. Demaitre, *Medieval Medicine*, 85–86, 96–97; Roy Porter, *Flesh in the Age of Reason* (New York: W. W. Norton, 2003), 46–47; William Buchan, *Domestic Medicine, or A Treatise for the Cure and Prevention of Diseases, by Regimen and Simple Medicines*. New edition (Halifax: Milner and Sowerby, 1859), 176.

9. Dewees, *A Treatise on the Physical and Medical Treatment of Children*, 310–319; Condie, *A Practical Treatise on the Diseases of Children*, xiv, 77.

10. Thomas E. Cone Jr., *History of American Pediatrics* (Boston: Little, Brown, 1979), 72–76; John Eberle, *A Treatise on the Diseases and Physical Education of Children* (Cincinnati, OH: Corey and Fairbank, 1833), 125–144; Calvert, *Children in the House*, 48–49; Sylvia Hoffert, *Private Matters: American Attitudes Toward Childbearing and Infant Nurture in the Urban North, 1800–1860* (Urbana: University of Illinois Press, 1989), 149; Lynne Curry, *Modern Mothers in the Heartland: Gender, Health, and Progress in Illinois, 1900–1930* (Columbus: The Ohio State University Press), 19.

11. Meckel, *Save the Babies*, 41; Rose A. Cheney, "Seasonal Aspects of Infant and Childhood Mortality: Philadelphia, 1865–1920," *Journal of Interdisciplinary History*, Volume 14, Number 3 (Winter 1984): 561–585; Samuel H. Preston and Michael R. Haines, *Fatal Years: Child Mortality in Late Nineteenth-Century America* (Princeton: Princeton University Press, 1991), 10.

12. Samuel Radbill, "The Pediatrics of Benjamin Rush," *Transactions and Studies of the College of Physicians of Philadelphia*, Volume 40, Number 3 (January 1973): 151–170; Cone, *History of American Pediatrics*, 44–45, 94. A rather more critical assessment of Rush can be found in Richard Harrison Shryock, *Medicine and Society in America 1660–1860* (New York: New York University Press, 1960).

13. Dewees, *A Treatise on the Physical and Medical Treatment of Children*, 416.

14. Dewees, *A Treatise on the Physical and Medical Treatment of Children*, 420–427.

15. Condie, *A Practical Treatise on the Diseases of Children*, 102–122; Alexandra Minna Stern and Howard Markel, "Introduction." In Alexandra Minna Stern and Howard Markel, editors, *Formative Years: Children's Health in the United States 1880–1920* (Ann Arbor: University of Michigan Press, 2002), 6–7. The French philosopher Michel Foucault used the notion of the "medical gaze" to describe a phenomenon of the early nineteenth century in which "doctors described what for centuries had remained below the threshold of the visible and the expressible." Physicians fundamentally transformed medical science by observing and naming diseases as discrete entities rather than as metaphorical states of humoral imbalance. *The Birth*

*of the Clinic: An Archaeology of Medical Perception.* A. M. Sheridan Smith, translator (New York: Vintage Books, 1994), xii.

16. Cone, *History of American Pediatrics*, 83; Meckel argues that monitoring and improving the feeding of infants remained the "single most important activity" of the new specialty of pediatrics for the remainder of the nineteenth century. *Save the Babies*, 45.

17. John Forsyth Meigs, *A Practical Treatise on the Diseases of Children* (Philadelphia: Lindsay and Blakiston, 1848); John R. Beck, *Essays on Infant Therapeutics* (New York: W.E. Dean, 1849), 11.

18. Cone, *History of American Pediatrics*, 73–83; Russell Viner, "Abraham Jacobi and the Origins of Scientific Pediatrics in America." In Stern and Markel, editors, *Formative Years*, 23–46.

19. Abraham Jacobi, "Address at the Twenty-Fifth Jubilee of the German Dispensary of New York." In A. Jacobi, *Miscellaneous Addresses and Writings*, Vol. VIII (New York: The Critic and Guide Company, 1909), 59–75; Meckel, *Save the Babies*, 46; Halpern, *American Pediatrics*, 56.

20. Regina Morantz-Sanchez, *Sympathy and Science: Women Physicians in American Medicine*. Reprinted (Chapel Hill: University of North Carolina Press, 2000), 184–202.

21. Job Lewis Smith, *A Treatise on the Diseases of Infancy and Children*. Second edition (Philadelphia: Henry C. Lee, 1872), 76; Cone, *History of American Pediatrics*, 103–104.

22. Stern and Markel, *Formative Years*, 3; Meckel, *Save the Babies*, 47; Sydney A. Halpern, *American Pediatrics: The Social Dynamics of Professionalism, 1880–1980* (Berkeley: University of California Press, 1988), 49.

23. Luther Emmett Holt, *The Diseases of Infancy and Childhood*. Second edition (New York: D. Appleton and Company, 1899), v–vi.

24. Jefferey P. Brosco, "Weight Charts and Well Child Care: When the Pediatrician Became the Expert in Child Health." In Alexandra Minna Stern and Howard Markel, editors, *Formative Years: Children's Health in the United States, 1880–2000* (Ann Arbor: University of Michigan Press, 2004), 91–120; Amanda M. Czerniawski, "From Average to Ideal: The Evolution of the Height and Weight Table in the United States, 1836–1943." *Social Science History*, Volume 31, Number 2 (Summer 2007): 273–296; Howard Markel, "For the Welfare of Children: The Origins of the Relationship Between U.S. Public Health Workers and Pediatricians." In Stern and Markel, editors, *Formative Years*, 47–65.

25. On medical education and licensing in the nineteenth-century U.S., see: Richard Harrison Shryock, *Medical Licensing in America, 1650–1965* (Baltimore: Johns Hopkins University Press, 1967); Paul Starr, *The Social Transformation of American Medicine* (New York: Basic Books, 1982); David A. Johnson and Humayun J. Chaudhry, *Medicine Licensing and Discipline in America* (Lanham, MD: Lexington Books, 2012); James C. Mohr: *Licensed to Practice: The Supreme Court Defines the American Medical Profession* (Baltimore: Johns Hopkins University Press, 2013).

# CHAPTER 3

# The Public Child

"Not long ago," says Dr. Annie S. Daniel, in the last report of the out-practice of the Infirmary for Women and Children, "we found in such an apartment five persons making cigars, including the mother. Two children were ill with diphtheria. Both parents attended to the children. They would syringe the nose of each child and, without washing their hands, return to the cigars."

In 1892, the social reformer Jacob A. Riis published the first edition of *The Children of the Poor*, a sequel to his best-selling book of two years earlier, *How the Other Half Lives*. Reflecting the broad scope of the nineteenth-century child welfare movement, Riis's work brought the public dimension of children's well-being to the forefront, including the risks posed by overcrowded conditions in tenement housing and the plight of "little toilers" engaged in factories and street trades. Further, *The Children of the Poor* reflected a particular view among social reformers, gaining currency at century's end, that framed child welfare in medicalized terms. To support his case for public involvement in children's well-being, Riis offered testimony from a physician whose credibility derived from her specialized clinical experience in caring for children's health. He focused readers' attention on two sympathetic young subjects suffering from diphtheria, a highly infectious disease known to be a leading cause of childhood mortality in the late nineteenth century. One particularly disturbing symptom of diphtheria

© The Author(s) 2019
L. Curry, *Religion, Law, and the Medical Neglect of Children in the United States, 1870–2000*, Palgrave Studies in the History of Childhood, https://doi.org/10.1007/978-3-030-24689-1_3

was the growth of a pseudomembrane in its victims' throats and nasal passages which, if left unattended, could obstruct a child's small airways, causing a slow and agonizing death. Although the overworked parents in Riis's scenario attempted to assuage their little ones' suffering by rinsing out their noses with a syringe, their apparent ignorance of diphtheria's highly contagious nature threatened to spread its horrors far beyond the walls of a single tenement dwelling, posing a danger to other people's children as well. Riis's vignette, while perhaps apocryphal, nevertheless broadcast a clear message: Reform efforts aimed at improving children's health must be informed by the latest views from medical science.[1]

For much of the nineteenth century, rates of infant and child mortality had remained staggeringly high, and the precise etiologies of virtually all childhood diseases were only vaguely understood. Parents, in partnership with healers of various kinds, addressed children's needs within the private household. By mid-century, however, medical theorists had begun taking a closer interest in investigating links between the private and public dimensions of children's health care. Cholera infantum, the diarrheal disease representing one of the most prolific killers of children under the age of five, had long been associated with both individual feeding practices and various elements of the larger environment, especially high summer temperatures and a lack of access to fresh air. But before the mid-nineteenth century such connections had been grounded in the speculative humoral theories that had long dominated western medical practices. Being naturally choleric in body and temperament, these theories posited, children required frequent adjustments in diet, clothing, and atmosphere for the purpose of regulating their bodies' tendency to overproduce yellow bile. Physicians such as Benjamin Rush had prescribed altering various environmental factors with the aim of bringing the child's body into a state of equilibrium. By the 1840s, however, medical science began to move away from the ancient humoral model and toward a paradigm that associated specific diseases with identifiable etiologies. Mid-century medical theorists turned their attention to investigating the possible role played by miasmas, or impure air, as major contributors to the spread of disease. Under the zymotic theory of contagion a number of childhood ailments, including cholera infantum, could be effectively addressed through large-scale environmental interventions such as draining stagnant water and trapping noxious sewer gasses. Thus efforts to improve individual children's health reached beyond the private household and became integrally connected to larger community health and sanitation efforts. At century's end, the public dimension of child welfare became even more pronounced with the epistemic revolution in medical theory brought about by bacteriology, which implicated new, previously unsuspected, vectors by which deadly diseases might spread. Drawing clear connections between the private and public dimensions of children's health, Jacob Riis's vignette promoted the view that the physical health of children required wider societal concern.[2]

By using compelling words and images to call attention to poor children's deprivations, Riis drew from an enduring cultural trope of suffering childhood that was well established by the time *The Children of the Poor* made its appearance. Antebellum social reformers, as well as writers of fiction, had created a powerful literary genre that had moved the sympathies of middle-class readers and helped to raise awareness of children's needs for physical care. American readers enthusiastically consumed child-centered stories, poetry, and fiction such as *Uncle Tom's Cabin*, Harriet Beecher Stowe's best-selling 1852 novel that featured one of the most celebrated child deathbed scenes in all of American literature. Like their fiction-writing counterparts, child welfare reformers also drew sympathetic portraits in an attempt to bridge the social gap between the lived experiences of poor and working-class children and the imaginative empathy of middle-class adults whose active engagement was needed to assuage their distress. Riis adapted the available trope of suffering childhood to convince his readers that the public must concern itself with children's health, a point he illuminated with sobering statistics on infant and childhood mortality from diseases that, like diphtheria, were known to be both deadly and contagious. For most of the 1800s, however, child welfare advocates had framed children's physical suffering primarily as a moral, rather than a medical, matter.[3]

Throughout the nineteenth century the injured and neglected bodies of children functioned as protean metaphors for expressing a wide range of social and political anxieties. Recent scholarship has explored the powerful cultural constructions that American writers and reformers used to reframe complex and abstract issues in terms that were direct, emotional, and personal. Karen Sánchez-Eppler notes that, while the sentimental rhetoric of childhood articulated a set of normative expectations for how Americans ought to live, portraits of suffering children brought into stark relief the ways that society failed to live up to those standards. Literary scholar Anna Mae Duane, for example, argues that both pro- and anti-slavery advocates drew upon such cultural conventions to justify their opposing causes. Although each side acknowledged the fact that slave children endured a great deal of physical hardship, they disagreed vehemently over which side was most capable of assuaging their plight. For abolitionists, enslaved children's lack of adequate nurture and care represented a compelling reason to destroy the institution itself. Duane asserts that, rather than putting forth human rights claims on behalf of parents who were enslaved, a strategy unlikely to gain traction among white northerners, abolitionists chose to "define the child as a subject who suffered mightily from a lack of loving care." In contrast, apologists for slavery countered that, far from perpetuating neglect, the institution allowed benevolent masters to provide food and shelter to thousands of children whose natural parents were innately incapable of addressing their needs. Ending slavery, they insisted, would cast these children to the same sad fate endured by the impoverished offspring of recent immigrants left to fend for themselves on the streets of northern industrial cities. Piercing through the political and economic discourses surrounding the abolition debate, the imagery of suffering childhood offered powerful "emotional leverage" that helped to force slavery into the national moral consciousness.[4]

Historians note that mid-nineteenth-century Americans used the term "cruelty" widely enough to encompass a variety of adult offenses against children, including drunkenness and moral laxity. Violence perpetrated against the bodies of children garnered considerable attention. The use of corporal punishment to discipline behavior, of course, was not a new phenomenon, and neither was its policing by the community. In colonial America, while the manner and severity of physical punishment had been largely left to parents' discretion, particularly that of fathers, authorities might intervene in extreme cases when physical correction clearly exceeded acceptable community standards. In 1669, for example, Mary Morey was brought before a Plymouth Colony court to answer for her "crewel, unnatural, and extreame" behavior in disciplining her son. While parental prerogatives remained important, a gradual evolution in cultural attitudes toward corporal punishment became evident as the tenets of Enlightenment child-rearing philosophy reached a mass audience through domestic advice literature aimed at a popular readership. Most influential was John Locke's treatise, *Some Thoughts Concerning Education*, a compendium of child-rearing advice he had given privately to friends that first appeared in published form in 1693.[5]

Much of what Locke addressed in these missives concerned the topic of discipline. He posited that, while violence may elicit immediate and superficial compliance, over the longer term it actually served to impede a child's moral development. For Locke, the ultimate objective of parenting was to produce an autonomous individual who would overcome his natural impulsivity and learn to "submit to his own Reason, when he is of an Age to make use of it." The philosopher urged that, rather than resorting to physical correction, adults should teach children to master their emotions and regulate their own behavior. Like most of his medical peers, the physician Locke regarded young children as innately choleric, or constitutionally prone to irritation and overexcitement. Children engaged in deliberately cruel and aggressive acts, however, by imitating behavior they observed in adults. Parents, he counseled, must "make Conscience not to mislead" their offspring by losing control of their own emotions and resorting to violence. While Locke saw a definite place for corporal punishment in education and training, he advised that harsh physical correction should be reserved for only the most egregious of infractions. Nearly a century after the publication of Locke's *Thoughts*, his rejection of capricious authority and stress on individuals' capacity for self-governance resonated in the political discourses opposing "tyranny" that permeated the early American republic. By 1850, Enlightenment perspectives on child-rearing, especially the view that childhood represented a critical formative stage in human character development, had made significant inroads into the daily domestic lives of middle-class Americans.[6]

Echoing the Enlightenment protest against authoritarian overreach, antebellum social reformers linked the physical abuse of children to a more generalized problem of violence in settings where subordinated individuals were kept confined and isolated, including prisons, mental asylums, and ships at sea. Within that broader context controversies arose over the excessive physical correction employed in newly established public schools. Although public, or common, schools proliferated in northern states, they lacked both professional standards and legal oversight. Education reformer Horace Mann argued that corporal punishment cruelly suppressed children's "natural exuberance" and led a successful campaign for statutory restrictions on the practice in Massachusetts. Similarly, antebellum temperance activists portrayed drunkenness as a crime perpetrated by brutish men toward the dependent children who had no choice but to live under their roofs. Samuel Chipman of the New York Temperance Society investigated that state's jails and workhouses, reporting that inmates' infractions frequently involved both drunkenness and domestic abuse, a finding that, for Chipman, offered incontrovertible proof that drinking liquor caused violent behavior. For temperance advocates, intoxication upended men's natural place as the loving heads and protectors of their households. Prohibiting the sale and distribution of alcohol would, they insisted, both ensure children's physical well-being and restore proper moral order in the home. And, because household harmony formed the foundation of social stability, adults' moral lapses into drunkenness and child abuse carried repercussions well beyond the walls of the private household.[7]

Antebellum reformers wrestled with another threat to children's physical well-being: parental neglect. New custodial institutions proliferated in response to the waning of the "placing out" system that had traditionally helped to ensure children remained under the watchful eyes of adults if their parents could not, or would not, properly care for them. Through both formal and informal arrangements, parents placed their children in other people's households to ensure they would receive at least minimal provision of food, clothing, and protection. The most unfortunate child neglect cases ended up alongside destitute adults in almshouses or workhouses, where minor children came under the supervision of local authorities. A stay in the almshouse was temporary by design, lest inmates become overly dependent on the community's largesse and fail to learn the habits of thrift and industry that would lead to their self-sufficiency. Children requiring longer-term care were therefore placed with families via formal indentures or apprenticeships in which a male head of household legally contracted with the overseers of the poor to provide for the child's physical care. Although the primary goal of these arrangements was to ensure community stability through the control of unsupervised youths, indentures arranged and administered by local authorities offered at least a modicum of assurance that a child's basic physical needs would be met by a responsible adult.[8]

But the severe economic and social dislocations set in motion by industrialization put unprecedented strains on the traditional placing-out system as the number of children whose parents were unable to care for them skyrocketed. In the 1830s and 1840s asylums designed to house the growing number of destitute children separately from adults proliferated throughout the country; by 1850 New York State alone had established twenty-seven such institutions. The zeal for social reform engendered by the Second Great Awakening inspired a wave of new private establishments that were founded by religious denominations and administered in coordination with secular authorities. Quakers, for example, established houses of refuge with the twin aims of sheltering and reforming child offenders who had been deemed criminally delinquent by local magistrates. Within the highly structured environment of the new asylums, Quaker leaders asserted, the "orphan, deserted, or misguided child" would be "shielded from the temptations of a sinful world" and also from the harmful influence of adult offenders—possibly including the child's own parents. Refuge administrators, in fact, viewed neglect by parents to be the main cause of children's deviant behavior, a perspective that permeated their fund-raising literature. The Boston Children's Friend Society, for example, appealed to donors by advertising its role in taking in children whom courts had removed from intemperate and uncaring parents in order to head off the "baleful influences" that would inevitably turn their sons and daughters into "pests to society" and "tenants of our prisons." Such entreaties made it clear that public indifference toward neglected children had ominous consequences for the larger community.[9]

Within a few decades, however, many reformers had become disillusioned with large-scale institutionalization as a solution to the plight of neglected children. Chronic underfunding and overcrowding, as well as an ethical discomfort with both the oppressive martial rigidity of the institutional environments and the severe physical punishments routinely inflicted on the small bodies of the inmates, caused a backlash from many child welfare advocates. In 1853 Charles Loring Brace founded the Children's Aid Society in New York City as an alternative to institutionalization. Brace's missionary zeal for child-saving stemmed from a calling he had received early in his vocation as a Congregationalist minister. He firmly believed that the neglected children of the poor properly belonged, not behind rigid asylum walls, but rather under the loving care and guidance they would receive in Protestant Christian homes. Like many of his contemporaries Brace saw only personal moral failing, not desperate circumstances precipitated by industrialization, in the behavior of parents who couldn't be "talked or driven into saving their own children" no matter how fervently reformers might try to persuade them. Notoriously, his aggressive interventions into the lives of poor families included transporting children of Irish and Italian immigrants away from the influence of their Roman Catholic parents—sometimes at considerable distances–and placing them with Protestant families where the "wild, neglected little outcasts of the streets" would receive proper care and guidance in "kind Christian homes." (Alarmed at the religious indoctrination that accompanied Protestant child-saving crusades, Catholic and Jewish communities organized their own efforts on behalf of poor families.) Brace held a view, common among nineteenth-century social reformers, that although the propensity toward crime and deviance appeared to be heritable, individual children could be rescued by altering their surroundings and influences. For Brace and his contemporaries, early intervention and loving, positive correction was the key to their salvation.[10]

Reformers concerned with the problem of neglect also believed that the work children performed, particularly in northern industrial cities, placed them beyond responsible adult oversight and exposed them to a range of physical and moral perils. Regardless of families' economic circumstances, or the coping strategies they used to keep their households intact, in reformers' eyes virtually all working children were neglected children. By the middle of the nineteenth century the well-regulated environment of the traditional apprenticeship system, in which children lived in their masters' households while they acquired skills preparing them for a trade or housewifery, had largely given way to the relative disorder of minors performing unskilled labor on industrial shop floors and city streets. Apprenticeships that did survive into the mid-nineteenth century more closely resembled adult wage labor in the free market. Young workers were increasingly likely to board away in lodging houses, for example, rather than living as full-time members of a master's household. One of Brace's earliest child-saving projects was to provide safe, clean, and inexpensive rooms to children who were employed in street trades, particularly the young boys who hawked newspapers in New York. Working in every part of the city, roaming freely at all hours of the day and night, newsboys embodied social reformers' worst fears about the exposure of unsupervised minors to physical and moral harm. What is more, time on the clock also meant time out of school, leaving child workers woefully unprepared to become self-sufficient and thereby dooming them to a lifetime of indolence and dependence on the community. Like physical abuse, for much of the nineteenth century, reformers framed child neglect as a fundamentally moral failing, the result of lazy and careless parents—especially fathers—who were unwilling to support their own offspring. Neglectful parents also failed to train their children in the virtues of obedience, self-control, and respect for authority, essential elements for maintaining order in the home and stability in the community. Appearing in both social reform literature and fictional portrayals, the ubiquitous character of the independent street waif—prematurely shrewd and perhaps even sexually precocious–stood as a powerful icon of childhood betrayed, particularly when juxtaposed against the imagery of children whose purity and innocence was safeguarded within the home. For city dwellers in industrializing America, large numbers of unsupervised urchins working and playing on busy streets provided daily and highly visible evidence that child neglect constituted a vital, and growing, public concern.[11]

In 1872 Brace published the first edition of his influential book, *The Dangerous Classes and Twenty Years' Work Among Them*, a lengthy and ambitious treatise offering an historical overview of suffering childhood extending back to ancient Rome. Brace began by depicting harsh and barbaric pagan practices which he then contrasted with the humanitarian influence that came about with the spread of Christianity. For the Congregationalist minister, Christianity's central doctrine was a belief in the "inestimable value of each immortal soul."; the souls of abused, neglected, and otherwise suffering children counted among the valued and deserved to be rescued most of all. Brace devoted a chapter of *The Dangerous Classes* to describing one of his early successes among an Italian immigrant community in New York's notorious Five Points district, an area well-known for its crime and gang violence. The narrative offers a clear illustration of how religiously motivated and influential child-savers like Brace understood the problem of child neglect, as well as the remedies they envisioned in the mid-nineteenth century. The chapter began with a description of the "degraded" state of the "little Italian organ-grinders" who were sent out by their parents to earn pennies on the dangerous streets of Five Points. The physical appearance of the young street musicians, Brace lamented, suggested they had descended from benighted ancestors who had "so mingled in North Italy with ancient Celtic blood, that their faces could hardly be distinguished from those of Irish poor children." But, despite the inherited propensity toward deviance he detected in their facial features, their "bright eyes" ultimately convinced Brace "there was mind in them" and thus they could still be salvaged. He set about establishing a day school where neighborhood children could receive a basic education and, even more importantly, proper Christian moral training. After an uncertain start made even rockier by clashes with a suspicious and interfering parish priest, eventually the community came to trust and appreciate the school. Brace corroborated his narrative of triumph with approving testimony from a Signor A. E. Cerqua, a local figure whom he assured readers was "a very intelligent Italian gentleman of education," and, most assuredly, "a Protestant." Writing many years later, Brace could point to the day school venture in Five Points as a template for future success should other reformers wish to replicate the experiment. Even so, after two decades of child-saving Brace believed that much work remained to be done. The miserable conditions still endured by thousands of children in New York and elsewhere, he maintained, represented nothing less than "one of the most threatening and painful phenomena of modern society." For Brace, addressing the plight of the neglected children of the poor constituted a religious imperative of the most urgent public dimensions.[12]

In the last quarter of the nineteenth century, a new kind of new anti-cruelty society drew public attention to the physical well-being of domestic animals as well as young children. Left unprotected by the adults who were charged with their care, these dependent beings were forced to fend for themselves under harsh conditions in urban industrial environments. Coordinating efforts and resources on behalf of animal as well as child welfare made practical sense in rapidly growing cities where formal social services were either scant or nonexistent. Organizations calling themselves "Humane Societies" divided their resources among a multiplicity of projects that included monitoring the care of livestock and horses, sheltering stray pets, and investigating cases of child abuse and neglect. In 1877, the founding of the American Humane Association brought this approach to social reform to the national stage. Historian Susan J. Pearson argues that, by drawing attention to physical hardships experienced by dependent animals and children alike, anti-cruelty advocates implicitly critiqued the early republic's liberal ethos of individualism and a minimal state, tenets no longer seen as functional in a society marked by massive economic and social dislocations. Although the new humane societies were private organizations, their anti-cruelty discourses helped to nourish a growing notion that government must step in when adults failed to provide for children's well-being. By the nineteenth century's end, social reformers began reframing child welfare as the child's right to receive a sustaining level of support for his or her physical needs. Gilded-Age humane societies therefore occupied a transitional space between antebellum reforms informed by religion and moral order and the secular, state-centered child welfare campaigns that would arise in the early twentieth century.[13]

In 1874, a nine-year-old child in New York City who had suffered severe abuse and neglect became the physical embodiment of child welfare's transition from the private to the public sphere. The case of Mary Ellen Wilson garnered unprecedented attention both within and beyond the city's limits. Newspapers covered her story extensively in the spring of that year. Later, in a reimagined form, the little girl's case came to serve as a creation myth for "discovery" of the problem of child abuse in the mid-nineteenth century, as well as for the New York Society for the Prevention of Cruelty to Children (SPCC). Founded by three prominent New York City philanthropists (Henry Bergh, Elbridge T. Gerry, and John D. Wright), the society's charter unreservedly proclaimed its mission to rescue "little children from the cruelty and demoralization which neglect, abandonment and improper treatment engender." Children, the charter's language indicated, deserved to have their physical needs addressed and, what is more, this organization would see that it happened. Other child protection advocates followed the SPCC's lead and by 1908 fifty-five societies had been founded throughout the United States. In reality, Mary Ellen Wilson was far from the first abused and neglected child to catch the attention of local authorities. Sadly, her case would not be the last. Only months after her plight entered the public's consciousness, for example, the *New York Times* reported the death of a four-year-old girl from injuries she received when her mother held her down on a hot stove, a tragedy that occurred just a few blocks from the apartment where Mary Ellen Wilson had endured her ordeal. Contrary to the SPCC's own publicity materials, this child's case did not represent a sudden and shocking "discovery" that child abuse and neglect existed. Rather, specific elements of little Mary Ellen's story came together to form a narrative made powerful by a profound rethinking of children's physical care taking place in the last quarter of the nineteenth century.[14]

The narrative began with the sympathetic figure of Marietta ("Etta") Wheeler, a woman whom press reports identified as a "sweet-faced" charity worker associated with a local Methodist church. Wheeler had been contacted by Margaret Bingham, a woman who rented a flat in her home to a couple named Mary and Francis Connolly. Bingham, along with other tenants of the house, noticed that a small child was locked up for hours in the Connollys' apartment while they were away. It seemed that she left the premises only to use the outdoor privy, appearing without shoes or stockings and wearing only the skimpiest of clothing even in extremely cold weather. If spotted outside of the flat, the little girl would "run like a hunted deer" back inside. Another couple, Charles and Mary Smith, lived in a flat that was adjacent to the Connollys' on the third floor of the house. Mary Smith, who was bedridden, told the charity worker that she often heard the little girl screaming and running back and forth inside the apartment next door. Disturbed by what she had learned from the tenants, Wheeler investigated further, using the pretense of asking Mary Connolly for help in looking after the ailing Mrs. Smith in order to gain entrance to the flat. Once inside, Wheeler "saw a pale, thin child" who was barefoot and clothed in tatters despite the cold December day. The charity worker estimated the little girl to be about five years old, although she would soon learn that the undersized child was in fact aged nine. Mary Ellen stood on a keg washing dishes in a bucket of water, and Wheeler observed that her arms and legs were severely bruised. Much to her horror, she also noticed a cowhide whip lying on a nearby table. Wheeler left that day but returned on several subsequent dates, ostensibly to discuss Mrs. Smith's care with Mary Connolly, but in reality to further investigate Mary Ellen's situation. Smith told Wheeler she continued to hear the child being abused by the Connollys, which convinced the charity worker that the little girl was in danger. Nevertheless she remained unsure of what action she should take, mindful against "arousing any suspicion lest the family disappear." Wheeler later wrote that during this time she "asked advice" from others but found that "no one could tell me what to do." While it isn't clear precisely whose advice she had sought (presumably law enforcement and her charitable organization, at a minimum), three months later she contacted Henry Bergh, a prominent philanthropist who in 1866 had founded the American Society for the Prevention of Cruelty to Animals (ASPCA).[15]

Significantly, Etta Wheeler was married to *New York Daily News* reporter Charles G. Wheeler, a fact that helps to explain the extensive interest the press took in the story, which clearly did not represent a singular case of apparent child abuse and neglect occurring in the city. What is more, the charity worker's intimate connection to the press reveals why journalists went beyond merely reporting the story and engaged in vigorous advocacy on Mary Ellen's behalf. By 1874, in fact, Henry Bergh already had been at the receiving end of press criticism. Local newspapers derided the philanthropist for coming to the aid of neglected animals while ignoring the needs of the city's poor. "The people who are so tender about a broken-winded horse," the *Daily News* had editorialized in 1867, "would find a wider field for their sympathy if they would pay a little more attention to the care of human beings." The *New York Telegram* was even more aggressive, snidely suggesting that "our model Christian, President Bergh, appears to have a hard time of it ... in his efforts to provide for the comfort of turtles, protect the interests of innocent calves, shield the ears of spaniels from the shears, and throw every person who is not as philanthropic and kind-hearted as himself into jail." Perhaps goaded by the unflattering press, in 1871 Bergh did attempt to intervene on behalf of an eight-year-old girl, applying successfully for a writ of habeas corpus to have the child removed from her abusive guardian. Appearing before the court, however, the frightened child denied she had been beaten and the judge, although finding the guardian guilty of cruelty, suspended the sentence and returned the child to her care because it seemed that the little girl had no other place to live. Following this failed attempt at child rescue the ASPCA director turned down subsequent appeals to use the organization's resources on behalf of abused and neglected children. While he may have preferred to distance himself from further personal failure, he undoubtedly also considered the prospect of losing public and financial support for the cause of animal welfare. Bergh stated publicly that, while cases involving children were no doubt distressing, they simply were "not in his particular line." Apparently, however, there was something about the story Bergh heard from Etta Wheeler that changed his mind. He asked the ASPCA's lawyer, Elbridge T. Gerry, to investigate the matter and report back to him. Convinced that the little girl's situation was dire, on April 8, 1874 Bergh petitioned the New York Supreme Court to have Mary Ellen removed from her home and brought before the court. Further, Bergh's petition also requested that Mary and Francis Connolly be placed under arrest.[16]

Judge Abraham R. Lawrence granted the writ and ordered the child to be brought to his courtroom immediately. At that point he also commenced proceedings to locate relatives with whom she might be placed. Transcripts from that hearing, which took place over several days, along with contemporary newspaper coverage provide most of the information that is known concerning Mary Ellen's early background. A number of key details remain murky. She was born either in 1863 or 1864 to a woman named Frances (Fannie) Connor and her husband, Thomas Wilson. The couple had met while both were employed at New York's St. Nicholas Hotel and had married in 1861 just prior to the onset of the Civil War. Thomas Wilson entered the army and died in 1864 in Virginia, whereupon his widow began receiving a pension of two dollars per week. Fannie Wilson decided to return to her job at the St. Nicholas Hotel and left her infant daughter with an acquaintance named Martha Score. Wilson gave Score her weekly widow's pension to pay for Mary Ellen's care, an arrangement the two women kept up for about a year until both Wilson and the money abruptly stopped showing up. In July, 1865 Martha Score took Mary Ellen to the New York Department of Charities and Corrections. The department's superintendent, George Kellock, placed the eighteen-month-old child in an almshouse located on Blackwell's Island, a spot of land in the middle of the East River where various prisons and hospitals had been sited since the eighteenth century. Mary Ellen remained in the almshouse for six months until February 1866, when she was indentured to Thomas and Mary McCormick. It is unclear why the couple, who had experienced the deaths of all three of their biological children, wanted to take a toddler into their home at that time. Mary McCormick claimed that her husband told her on numerous occasions that he was the child's natural father and, what is more, he had fathered two additional children with Fannie Wilson. Thomas McCormick had also called Wilson "a good for nothing" and had insisted she was alive and living "somewhere down town" even though her baby remained languishing in the almshouse. Superintendent Kellock handed over Mary Ellen to the McCormicks on the basis of a single character reference, from a man whom the couple claimed was their family physician. (Subsequently, Judge Abraham Lawrence was unable to locate any such doctor.) Although the McCormicks took the child home, several months elapsed before an official contract was drawn up and signed. Within a year Thomas McCormick died and his widow married Francis Connolly. Mary Ellen Wilson continued to live with Francis and Mary Connolly, neither of whom had clear legal claims to her custody, under nightmarish circumstances for the next six years.[17]

On April 10, 1874 Mary Ellen was forcibly removed from the Connollys' flat by ASPCA agent Alonzo S. Evans, accompanied by two police detectives. Making a dramatic entrance in Judge Lawrence's chambers, the agent carried the tiny girl wrapped in a blanket and clutching a peppermint stick, which Evans had stopped to purchase for her on the way to the courthouse. Evans told the judge that, when the three men had entered the apartment, Mary Connolly had verbally abused them while Mary Ellen cowered in a corner, covering her face with her hands. The accompanying police detectives added the detail that Connolly had behaved in a vulgar manner toward Evans, crudely propositioning the young agent. Judge Lawrence next heard from Mary Ellen herself who, speaking through her ASPCA counsel (the judge did not allow the child to be sworn in under oath), provided a disturbing account of the violence and neglect she had been subjected to by Mary Connolly, whom she referred to as "mamma." Mary Ellen did not know her age. She had never attended school. She had never played with, nor even spoken to, another child. Currently clad in a skimpy calico dress, she could not remember ever wearing stockings and could recall having only one pair of shoes. She had never been held or kissed. In addition to being thrashed with the cowhide whip and burned with an iron, she recently had been stabbed in the forehead with scissors by Mary Connolly, who had become enraged that the child held a quilt incorrectly while Connolly attempted to pick out the stitching. Mary Ellen told the court that such inexplicably brutal attacks by her mamma occurred on a daily basis.[18]

Extensive press coverage brought spectators to the court as the shocking story continued to unfold the next day. "Humane ladies and gentlemen," the *New York Times* asserted, had become "interested in the fate of the child" and taken up her cause. Having spent the night in the care of a police matron Mary Ellen now sat quietly in the courtroom, dressed in new clothing and looking at a picture book, when Connolly made her first appearance before Judge Lawrence. In a "voluble" manner, the woman responded to the disturbing allegations that had been made against her on the previous day. Connolly explained she did not allow Mary Ellen to play outside on the street because she feared the little girl would "become contaminated by the other children" whom, she claimed, swore and behaved badly. She insisted that, despite the murky documentation of the arrangement between Superintendent Kellock and the McCormicks, Mary Ellen's indenture had been legally valid. Connolly adamantly maintained she had never received money in exchange for the little girl's care. She had taught Mary Ellen "that there is a God, and what it is to lie," a duty specified under the terms of the indenture. (That admission, incidentally, qualified the nine-year-old child to give sworn testimony against Connolly at her subsequent criminal trial.) The woman did admit that, while their arrangement required her to report annually to the Commissioners of Charities and Corrections, she had felt it necessary to comply only in the first two years because the commissioner "did not seem to care." Connolly became particularly agitated when questioned about the little girl's lack of appropriate clothing. She responded by defensively denouncing the proceedings as "meddlesome" and "an interference by people who did not know what they were doing." After hearing from a number of witnesses, including the Connollys' suspicious neighbors, the former caregiver Mary Score, and the charity superintendent George Kellock, Judge Lawrence closed the hearing and ordered the permanent removal of the child from the Connollys' custody. Naming himself as Mary Ellen's legal guardian, he placed her at the Sheltering Arms, a refuge for "fallen" young women run by the Episcopal Church. Despite the seeming unsuitability of such an arrangement for this child, Mary Ellen remained there for about eight months before Judge Lawrence transferred her to another institution in the city, the Woman's Aid Society and Home for Friendless Girls. Finally, in June, 1875, he granted custody of Mary Ellen to the charity worker Etta Wheeler, who took the child to live with her sister in Ogden, a small town in western New York State.[19]

Mary Ellen's physical appearance received an inordinate amount of attention in the press coverage of her case. "She is a bright little girl," noted the *New York Times*, "with features indicating unusual mental capacity, but with a care-worn, stunted, and prematurely aged look." Scrutinizing her body looking for signs of abuse and neglect, the reporter opined that "her apparent condition of health, as well as her scanty wardrobe, indicated that no change of custody or condition could be much for the worse" than the situation she had already endured in the Connolly home. The *Tribune* was even less equivocal, asserting that the child appeared "stunted in growth" and was clad in an "apology for a dress." As she was being carried into Judge Lawrence's chambers in the arms of agent Evans, Mary Ellen's "little pinched white face stretched out [from the folds of the blanket], and the small brown eyes peered forth in wonder." The child's hands and feet appeared very rough from exposure, and her body bore numerous observable injuries validating her account of abuse. Even more chilling, a disfiguring gash extended from her forehead to her ear, only just missing her left eye, a grim testament to the recent scissors attack by Mary Connolly. (Many years later Mary Ellen's daughters recalled the scar still surrounding their mother's eye.) On the second day of the hearing, the police matron testified that Mary Ellen's body was so dirty it had been necessary to bathe her three times. Her hair, which was infested with lice, appeared to never have been combed at all. What is more, she had observed distinctive red marks on the child's hip, arm, and temple and, when asked, Mary Ellen confirmed that Connolly had struck her with a cowhide whip. When Judge Lawrence announced his intention to seek out any living relatives of the child before making a final disposition as to her custody, the *Times* embellished the narrative with a touch of romance and mystery, speculating that despite her present physical condition "the intelligent and refined appearance of the child, tends to the conclusion that she is the child of parents of some prominence in society who for whatever reason have abandoned her to her present undeserved state." As if to highlight Mary Ellen's potential for rehabilitation given proper care and attention, the *Tribune* made note of the "pleasing and childlike" smile the girl gave Etta Wheeler upon spotting the charity worker in the courtroom. According to rather dubious press reports, Judge Lawrence was being besieged by both local and distant offers to adopt the child.[20]

Only a few weeks after the well-publicized custody hearing, Mary Ellen came under the glare of the public spotlight once again, this time at the criminal trial of Mary Connolly, who had been indicted by a grand jury on several charges of battery and felonious assault. The *New York Herald* noted a nearly miraculous improvement in the child's physical appearance. She was now, the paper noted, clean and "tastefully dressed," a change that made her look "more like the petted daughter of wealthy parents than a tenement house 'waif.'" The *Times* concurred with the extraordinary alteration in Mary Ellen's appearance, observing that the "interesting looking child" now seemed to be "years younger" and nearly unrecognizable from her initial appearance in Judge Lawrence's court. Such a profound physical transformation, the happy result of proper attendance to a child's physical well-being, struck a hopeful and redemptive note in the emerging narrative of Mary Ellen Wilson's experience. Long after the conclusion of her case, contrasting images of the suffering and the recovering child appeared regularly in SPCC publicity materials. More widely, her likeness was reproduced in magazines that featured stories and poems recounting her story and her photograph was displayed at exhibitions promoting the work of child protective organizations. The little girl's image even graced the covers of sheet music for popular songs.[21]

What is truly noteworthy about the narrative that emerged from Mary Ellen Wilson's case is the public meaning that so quickly became transcribed onto the facts of the case. Unlike earlier reform discourses surrounding childhood abuse and neglect, press coverage did not present this young girl as a "pest" of the "dangerous classes" whose privations posed a threat to community safety and moral order. Instead, the reportage highlighted the fact that a gross injustice had been perpetrated upon a vulnerable and dependent being; this child, the narrative asserted unequivocally, deserved better. Poignant details that reporters inserted into the accounts of the case clearly established Mary Ellen as an authentic child, not a sly and menacing proto-criminal prematurely hardened into adulthood. Upon facing her abuser in Judge Lawrence's chambers, Mary Ellen reportedly gave Mary Connolly a simple and artless greeting: "Good morning, mamma. I have got new clothes." Called to testify at Connolly's criminal trial some weeks later, the nine-year-old took the stand in yet another public accounting of her experiences. While it was not uncommon for children to act as legal witnesses in nineteenth-century criminal trials (and the previous court had established she was fully capable of understanding the meaning of her sworn oath to tell the truth), the press was particularly sympathetic to the hardship of the child's nerve-wracking ordeal. "At first she answered the questions put to her readily," the *New York Times* explained, "but soon [she] became frightened and gave way to sobs and tears." Fortunately, after receiving "kind words" of encouragement from the district attorney, the little witness recovered her composure and "intelligently detailed the story of her ill-treatment" to the court. It was convincing testimony. After deliberating for only twenty minutes, the jury convicted Mary Connolly of assault and Judge John K. Hackett sentenced her to one year at hard labor. In pronouncing the stiff sentence Judge Hackett remarked that, by assigning the maximum penalty allowed to him under the law, he intended to send a "warning to others" that such gross mistreatment of a child would not be tolerated. Adults were not free to act with impunity in their behavior toward young and vulnerable dependents in their household; courts could—and would—step in to protect children against gratuitous physical pain and suffering. Ultimately, the moral lesson to be drawn from the story of Mary Ellen Wilson was not that she posed a risk to the community's order, but rather that the abuse and neglect inflicted upon her small body offended public decency and deserved the severest sanction of the law.[22]

Scholars of childhood have noted a constellation of social and cultural changes that, taken together, reflect a new and unprecedented value placed upon the child's body in the last half of the nineteenth century. As Vivian A. Zelizer convincingly argued, the sentimental importance of children burgeoned as their economic contribution to the household declined, a phenomenon that spread gradually from middle- to working-class families. In mid-century, for example, middle-class parents adopted more elaborate funerary and mourning practices, raising the cultural standards by which to demonstrate proper respect for a lost child's memory. Mortuary photographs became customary as a way for parents to retain a beloved physical likeness long after the burial had taken place. By the 1890s, working-class parents bought special accident insurance policies that allowed them to meet the more elaborate—and more expensive—expectations for what constituted a "decent" burial should they lose a child. Images of living children became highly prized commodities as well. Scholar Josephine Gear noted that formally posed studio portraits offered a way for middle-class parents to present their children to family and community members, a privilege once reserved to elites who exhibited paintings of their offspring. Parents, particularly mothers, framed and displayed a child's photograph on a mantle or piano where it could be easily seen (and admired) by visitors to the home. Looking at pictures of babies and young children in family albums became a shared social pastime as well. Whether they appeared in family photographs or in the elaborate and colorful illustrations that now graced the pages of mass circulation magazines, images of children proved so popular they were routinely used to advertise a wide range of commercial products, from soap to patent medicines. Damaged bodies, by contrast, marked a betrayal of sentimentalized childhood and thus served as potent symbols of social injustice and moral offense. Historian James D. Schmidt observed that reformers seeking to abolish child labor regularly portrayed industrial America's "little toilers" as stooped, wizened, and deformed in appearance.[23]

The new emphasis on the intrinsic value of the child's body raised expectations for adults who were entrusted with the physical care of children. In 1873 pediatrics pioneer Abraham Jacobi published *Infant Diet*, the first substantial medical text dedicated exclusively to the topic of feeding that brought Jacobi's work on children's health to national attention. Never one to simply "let nature take its course," Jacobi counseled intensive and active monitoring of children's physical states, by both physicians and parents. The following year (when the public became aware of the severe abuse and neglect endured by Mary Ellen Wilson) Abraham Jacobi's wife, the physician and medical educator Mary Putnam Jacobi, adapted *Infant Diet* for a popular readership. In the new edition's introduction Putnam Jacobi asserted that, even without formal medical training, any mother was capable of understanding "the general plan of her child's life, its future course, and the accidents that beset it." Once such understanding was established, the logic implied, a responsible mother would naturally adapt her own child-rearing practices to comport with physicians' views. Putnam Jacobi intended the new edition to "set forth some of the more assured facts in the possession of science" regarding the "chemical changes that take place in the infant economy during the process of nutrition" so that mothers could make intelligent decisions about feeding their children. Informed by medical science, particularly the new field of pediatrics, new and higher standards for children's physical well-being were working their way to a broader public audience. With the founding of the American Pediatric Society in 1888 regular physicians took a definitive step in establishing a larger role for themselves as authorities in child welfare. In 1896, Luther Emmett Holt's *Diseases of Infancy and Childhood* emphasized the practice of routinely weighing and measuring children's bodies as a scientific, ostensibly objective, way to monitor their overall health status. The child's physical appearance had taken on new scientific, as well as social and cultural, significance.[24]

The following year, the National Congress of Mothers held its first meeting in Washington, DC, designed as a forum to bring together the "mothers of the land" who were "concerned with questions most vital to the welfare of their children." The newly formed Mothers' Congress joined a host of national-level associations such as the General Federation of Women's Clubs in harnessing middle-class women's activism in the service of advancing child welfare, defined in terms that stretched well beyond the preservation of moral order. Its first meeting covered a wide range of topics assumed to be of interest to modern mothers including kindergartens, playgrounds, nature studies, music, literature, and heredity. The Congress also addressed a diverse universe of maternal experiences such as "primitive motherhood," "mothers of the submerged world," "the Hebrew home," and "the Afro-American mother." Several speakers focused on the topic of children as unique physical entities whose specialized needs for care required serious study and diligence on the part of their caregivers. In "Dietetics," for example, Louise E. Hogan made it clear that mothers' responsibilities required them to become familiar with the latest, decidedly higher, standards that were now being set by pediatricians and by which their own children would be measured. "Dr. Jacobi says good food for a baby does not mean one which simply does not kill," she explained to her audience. "It is one that permits a child to grow up healthy and strong." What is more, the informed vigilance expected in infant care extended throughout the entire period of childhood. "If we will fully appreciate our whole duty to our children," Hogan continued, "we will avoid all uncertain methods and consider carefully, and estimate at its full importance, every point relating to the feeding of a child from infancy to adolescence." In a speech entitled "Mother's Relation to the Sound Physical Development of Her Child," Congress member A. Jennesse Miller carried the banner further, calling upon women's clubs to take up the scientific study of nutrition, physiology, and child development in order to properly attend to their children's physical well-being. "Disease is a crime," Miller stated unequivocally, and one that apparently would no longer be tolerated.[25]

Like proper growth and nutrition, treatable conditions afflicting a child's body also became a focus of intense concern among child welfare advocates. Volunteers with the Massachusetts Society for the Prevention of Cruelty to Children, for example, noted in their official reports a litany of infected sores, lice, ringworm, and eye and ear maladies that plagued the bodies of the neglected children whose cases they investigated. Dealing with common childhood ailments was not, of course, a new adult responsibility. Parents, particularly mothers, had traditionally diagnosed ailments among members of their households and selected from among a variety of available therapeutic options in treating them. In the late nineteenth century, however, new standards for children's physical care expected adults to align their therapeutic choices with the latest views promoted by physicians who were trained in regular medicine. An essential part of caregivers' responsibility was determining the point at which their own ministrations were insufficient and the services of medical doctors would be required. Increasingly, seeking professional medical care fell within an expanding rubric of duties that adults owed to children, regardless of their therapeutic preferences or their financial means. Failure to do so now constituted medical neglect—an adult infraction that had not been conceivable when regular medical science had little to offer in the way of preventing and treating childhood disease and death, but which now represented a matter of public concern. Further, as new discoveries from the laboratory sciences began to reshape the understanding of disease transmission, the link between the private and public dimensions of caring for children's bodies came ever more sharply into focus. Parents who allowed treatable illnesses and injuries to go unaddressed endangered the bodies of their own children and threatened those of other people's children as well. At the close of the nineteenth century, reformers reimagined the trope of suffering childhood to include children whose needs for professional medical attention went unaddressed by adults. Increasingly, they framed medical care as a child's right.[26]

## NOTES

1. Jacob Riis, *The Children of the Poor* (New York: Charles Scribner's Sons, 1908), 99. On Riis's construction of social reform through prose and imagery see David Leviatin, "Part One Introduction: Framing the Poor—The Irresistibility of *How the Other Half Lives*." In Jacob A. Riis, *How the Other Half Lives* (Boston: Bedford Books/St. Martin's Press, 2011), 1–50; Keith Gandall, *The Virtues of the Vicious: Jacob Riis, Stephen Crane, and the Spectacle of the Slum* (New York: Oxford University Press, 1997).
2. Richard A. Meckel, *Save the Babies: American Public Health Reform and the Prevention of Infant Mortality, 1850–1929* (Baltimore: Johns Hopkins University Press, 1990), 43.
3. Anna Mae Duane notes that the sentimental depiction of Little Eva's ordeal carried powerful resonances in a young republic still wrestling with

profound tensions over how to reconcile dichotomies such as dependence versus autonomy and vulnerability versus power—a legacy deeply embedded in its colonial experience. *Suffering Childhood in Early America: Violence, Race, and the Making of the Child Victim* (Athens: University of Georgia Press, 2010), 5–18. On the parallel movement in nineteenth-century Great Britain see Galia Benziman, *Narratives of Child Neglect in Romantic and Victorian Culture* (New York: Palgrave Macmillan, 2012).

4. Sánchez-Eppler, *Dependent States*, xxiii; Duane, *Suffering Childhood*, 125–164.

5. John Demos, *A Little Commonwealth: Family Life in Plymouth Colony*. Second edition (New York: Oxford University Press 2000), 100–106.

6. Historian Hugh Cunningham asserted that Locke addressed corporal punishment "obsessively." *Children and Childhood in Western Society Since 1500*. Second edition (Harlow, UK: Pearson Education Limited, 2005), 58–62. On the popularization of Locke's ideas in the early American republic see Jay Fliegelman, *Prodigals and Pilgrims: The American Revolution Against Patriarchal Authority 1750–1800* (Cambridge: Cambridge University Press, 1982).

7. Myra C. Glenn, *Campaigns Against Corporal Punishment: Prisoners, Sailors, Women, and Children in Antebellum America* (Albany: State University of New York Press, 1984), 18–19; Elizabeth Pleck, *Domestic Tyranny: The Making of American Social Policy Against Family Violence from Colonial Times to the Present* (New York: Oxford University Press, 1987), 48; Karen Sánchez-Eppler, *Dependent States: The Child's Part in Nineteenth-Century American Culture* (Chicago: University of Chicago Press, 2005), 75–81; and Caroline F. Lavender, *Cradle of Liberty: Rae, the Child, and National Belonging from Thomas Jefferson to W.E.B. DuBois* (Durham, NC: Duke University Press, 2006), 78–110.

8. David J. Rothman, *The Discovery of the Asylum: Social Order and Disorder in the New Republic* (New York: Little, Brown, and Company, 1990), 3–56; John E. Murray, "Bound by Charity: The Abandoned Children of Late Eighteenth-Century Charleston." In Billy G. Smith, editor, *Down and Out in Early America* (University Park, PA: Pennsylvania State University Press, 2004), 213–232; and Ruth Wallis Herndon and John E. Murray, editors, *Children Bound to Labor: The Pauper Apprentice System in Early America* (Ithaca: Cornell University Press, 2009).

9. LeRoy Ashby, *Endangered Children: Dependency, Neglect, and Abuse in American History* (New York: Twayne Publishers, 1997), 25, 48; Rothman, *The Discovery of the Asylum*, 77, 206–236.

10. In 1863 Brace published *The Races of the Old World: An Ethnology*, a sweeping treatise in which he ordered ethnic groups as he perceived them in a ranking of human progress. Charles L. Brace, *The Races of the Old World: A Manual of Ethnology* (New York: Charles Scribner, 1863).

11. Ashby, *Endangered Children*, 55; Steven Mintz, *Huck's Raft: A History of American Childhood* (Cambridge, MA: Harvard University Press, 2006), 138; James D. Schmidt, "'Restless Movements Characteristic of Childhood': The Legal Construction of Child Labor in Nineteenth-Century Massachusetts," *Law and History Review*, Volume 23, Number 2 (Summer 2005): 315–350; and James D. Schmidt, *Industrial Violence and the Legal Origins of Child Labor* (New York: Cambridge University Press, 2010), 47–57.

12. Charles Loring Brace, *The Dangerous Classes and Twenty Years Work Among Them.* Third edition (New York: Wynkoop and Hallenbeck, 1880), 13–24, 194–211. Brace's use of Cerqua's authenticating testimony is discussed in Keith Gandall, *The Virtues of the Vicious*, 35–36.

13. Susan J. Pearson, *The Rights of the Defenseless: Protecting Animals and Children in Gilded Age America* (Chicago: University of Chicago Press, 2011), 1–20.

14. Ashby, *Endangered Children*, 56–59; "History," New York Society for the Prevention of Cruelty to Children, https://www.nyspcc.org/about-the-new-york-society-for-the-prevention-of-cruelty-to-children/history/; Lela B. Costin, "Unraveling the Mary Ellen Legend: Origins of the 'Cruelty' Movement," *Social Service Review*, Volume 65, Number 2 (June 1991): 203–223; Mintz, *Huck's Raft*, 167–170; "A Revolting Tragedy: A Child Roasted to Death on a Stove by Its Mother," *New York Times* (November 25, 1874): 2.

15. Eric A. Shelman and Stephen Lazoritz, editors, *The Mary Ellen Wilson Child Abuse Case and the Beginning of Children's Rights in 19th Century America* (Jefferson, NC: McFarland and Company, 2005), 12–19, 160–166.

16. Shelman and Lazoritz, *The Mary Ellen Wilson Child Abuse Case*, 55–62, 112–113; Costin, "Unraveling the Mary Ellen Legend," 205–206.

17. New York State Supreme Court, Historical Society of the New York Courts, http://www.nycourts.gov/history/legal-history-new-york/history-legal-bench-supreme-court.html; Shelman and Lazoritz, *The Mary Ellen Wilson Child Abuse Case*, 166–186; "Mr. Bergh Enlarging His Sphere of Influence," *New York Times* (April 10, 1874): 8; and "The Mission of Humanity," *New York Times* (April 11, 1874): 2.

18. "A Child's Suffering," *New York Tribune* (April 11, 1874): 5; "The Mission of Humanity," 12; "Mary Ellen Wilson," *New York Times* (April 12, 1874): 12; and "Cruelty to a Child," *New York Tribune* (April 12, 1874): 2.

19. "Terrible Cruelty to a Child," 2; "Cruelty to a Child," 2. Mary Ellen Wilson continued to live in rural New York until her death in 1956 at the age of ninety-two. Shelman and Lazoritz, *The Mary Ellen Wilson Child Abuse Case*, 187–220.

20. "Mr. Bergh Enlarging His Sphere of Influence," 8; "Terrible Cruelty to a Child," *New York Tribune* (April 10, 1874): 2; Shelman and Lazoritz, *The Mary Ellen Wilson Child Abuse Case*, 166–169.

21. "Court of General Sessions," *New York Herald* (April 28, 1874): 11; "Mary Ellen Wilson," 12; and Pearson, *The Rights of the Defenseless*, 10–11.

22. "Mary Ellen Wilson," *New York Times* (April 28, 1874): 8; "Cruelty to a Child," 2.

23. Sánchez-Eppler, *Dependent States*, 101–149; Vivian A. Zelizer, *Pricing the Priceless Child: The Changing Social Value of Children* (New York: Basic Books, 1985), 32, 113–137; Josephine Gear, "The Baby's Picture: Woman as Image Maker in Small-Town America," *Feminist Studies*, Volume 13, Number 2 (Summer 1987): 419–442; and Schmidt, *Industrial Violence*, 63–64.

24. Richard A. Meckel, *Save the Babies: American Public Health Reform and the Prevention of Infant Mortality, 1850–1929* (Baltimore: Johns Hopkins University Press, 1990), 49–51; A. Jacobi, *Infant Diet*. Revised, Enlarged, and Adapted to Public Use by Mary Putnam Jacobi (New York: G. P. Putnam's Sons, 1874), v, 9; and Rhoda Truax, *The Doctors Jacobi* (Boston: Little, Brown, and Company, 1952), 174.

25. National Congress of Mothers, *The Work and Words of the First National Congress of Mothers* (New York: D. Appleton, 1897), vii, 111, 121.

26. Linda Gordon, *Heroes of Their Own Lives: The Politics and History of Family Violence* (New York: Penguin Books, 1988), 127–129.

# CHAPTER 4

# The Metaphysical Child

If a child comes from God it cannot be mortal and material; it must be immortal and spiritual.[1]

In 1875 Mary Baker Glover laid out the basic tenets of a metaphysical paradigm in a self-published treatise entitled *Science and Health with Key to the Scriptures*. Four years later, the recently remarried Mary Baker Eddy formally institutionalized her ideas as the First Church of Christ, Scientist, and the treatise, along with the Christian Bible, became the new religion's foundational text. The new church, which was headquartered in Lynn, Massachusetts, proliferated rapidly throughout the United States, becoming the fastest growing religion in American history. Healing the sick formed the core of the new religion, framed in terms of the founder's distinctive ideas about the causes and meaning of human suffering. Eddy insisted the tenets of the new religion had been demonstrated through Jesus's own ministrations to the sick but were subsequently forgotten until she herself had recently rediscovered them. The power to heal, she wrote, was "lost sight of, and must again be spiritually discerned; and it must be demonstrated (according to Christ's command) with signs following." Prior to the publication of *Science and Health*, Christian leaders commonly addressed the topic of bodily health in their writings and sermons. Among the most

© The Author(s) 2019
L. Curry, *Religion, Law, and the Medical Neglect of Children in the United States, 1870–2000*,
Palgrave Studies in the History of Childhood,
https://doi.org/10.1007/978-3-030-24689-1_4

influential published works was *Primitive Physick*, the eighteenth-century treatise in which Methodism's founder John Wesley affirmed the wisdom of the Creator by asserting the essential interconnectedness of medicine and religion. Following the Second Great Awakening, several new Protestant sects in the United States such as the Seventh-Day Adventism linked physical well-being to spiritual piety. Christian Science, however, stood in stark contrast to both traditional and recent religious doctrines because its founder expressly denied the material reality of sickness and, indeed, of the human body itself. Appearing in the last quarter of the nineteenth century, Christian Science marked a clear contrast to secular society's increasing recognition of children as distinctive biological entities with unique physical needs and requirements for care, a change expressed through a number of social and cultural trends that placed unprecedented importance on the body of the child.[2]

Eddy structured her metaphysical doctrine as follows: The material world, which she called Matter, was illusory. The only reality was the Divine Mind or God. Scripture revealed that God had created human beings in his own image. Therefore, because Divine Mind was both perfect and all-powerful, human disease and death could not possibly exist. "Erring, sick, and dying men are not the likeness of the perfect and eternal Mind," Eddy asserted in *Science and Health*. Humans experienced suffering only because they failed to comprehend their own true natures as the manifestations of God's wisdom and perfection. Eddy referred to the belief that one was sick as Error; a person's "claim" of illness was always false and reflected a limited and flawed understanding of the divine. Physical healing therefore entailed a process by which the sufferer mentally corrected Error—the mistaken belief that he or she was ill—and replaced it with Truth—knowledge that one's illness did not exist. As her biographer Stephen Gottschalk explained, in Christian Science healing happened "not through blind faith or miraculous divine intervention, but through understanding more of God's love and the supremacy of his power." This result was achieved primarily through reading scripture and Eddy's own treatise, *Science and Health with Key to the Scriptures*. Unlike the ecstatic rites used in other faith-healing sects, Christian Science employed abstract, intellectualized arguments and urged the repression of emotional impulses, particularly fearful responses to pain, that Eddy believed lay at the root of human suffering.[3]

In a glossary appended to *Science and Health* she defined the term "children" in distinctly non-corporeal terms:

Life, Truth, and Love's spiritual thoughts and representatives; sensual and mortal beliefs, counterfeits of creation, whose better originals are God's thoughts, not in embryo, but in maturity; material suppositions of life, substance, and intelligence, opposed to the Science of Being.

Earthly children, then, represented "counterfeits" or reproductions of their true forms, which consisted of God's thoughts, i.e., the "Science of Being." By extension, children's physical ailments were also illusory, just as they were for adults. Taken to its logical extreme, Eddy's teaching raised disturbing questions about adults' responsibilities to provide medical assistance when children became sick or injured. The first edition of *Science and Health* appeared in 1875, just one year after Mary Ellen Wilson's ordeal of abuse and neglect captivated the public's attention, a reflection of a new social ethos in which substantial numbers of Americans concerned themselves with the physical well-being of children. What is more, medical neglect itself had emerged as a new and distinctive category of infraction perpetrated by adults who failed to attend to children's health care needs. Lack of medical attention, particularly for conditions that had become treatable, came under the scrutiny of child protective workers and, increasingly, by courts as well, rendering parental decisions in their children's health care into matters of public, and not merely private, concern. By contrast, Eddy counseled her followers that their children's physical ailments were merely illusory. "That mother is not a Christian Scientist, and her affections need better aids," she wrote in 1889, "who says to her child: 'You look sick' or 'You look tired'; 'You need rest' or 'You need medicine.'" Eddy required her followers to make an unequivocal choice between medicine and Christian Science; there could be no compromise.[4]

Although she revised *Science and Health* continually, publishing over four hundred editions by 1907, Eddy framed her tenets as immutable laws not subject to alteration by evidence from the material world. "No human tongue or pen has suggested the contents of 'Science and Health,'" she assured her readers, "nor can tongue or pen ever overthrow it." Importantly, Eddy insisted that all other healing practices were fundamentally incompatible with Christian Science. Her rejection was not limited to regular medicine, however. Because they were based in material suppositions about the human body she regarded alternative healing sects, including homeopathy which was grounded in a pharmacopeia of medicinal compounds (a school that Eddy herself had once dabbled in but ultimately rejected), to be equally complicit in causing rather than curing human sickness. "My experience has proven to me the fallacy of the medical art," she asserted. "When Christianity overcomes *Materia medica*, and replaces faith in drugs with faith in God, sickness will disappear." As long as physicians had little to offer in the way of actually curing diseases, a wide range of therapeutic regimes enjoyed more or less equal chances of bringing relief to the ailing. Indeed, the tradition of restoring humoral balance via harsh remedies such as blistering, bleeding, and purging doubtlessly rendered many alternatives to regular medicine attractive to people already enduring physical distress. No less eminent a physician as Benjamin Rush had advocated bleeding to remediate fevers, even for infants (including his own) in the early American republic. By the late nineteenth century, however, new evidence being gathered in the material world was radically transforming medical understandings of disease, including the deadly childhood scourges of cholera infantum and diphtheria that still sickened and killed tens of thousands of children every year. As it gained influence among both regular physicians and the public at large, the new science of bacteriology posed a direct challenge to Eddy's metaphysical views. By the century's end, reconciling regular medicine with her own teachings became increasingly problematic for the founder of Christian Science, forcing her to rethink and revise several of the new religion's core tenets after the church became embroiled in legal difficulties. The growing disjuncture between physical and metaphysical healing also caused a profound dilemma for Christian Scientist parents who, while remaining steadfast in their religious commitment, risked criminal prosecution when their children died without receiving medical attention.[5]

Contrary to her own characterization of the origins of Christian Science, Eddy's creation of the metaphysical child did not arise in an intellectual vacuum. Throughout the nineteenth century, in fact, a broad swath of the American public searched for correspondences between the material and spiritual worlds, inspiring myriad new movements that combined, in varying proportions, the secular and the religious. While the New England Transcendentalists shocked many orthodox Protestant leaders by conflating divinity and nature, popular attractions such as séances and spirit photography suggested to many Americans that the boundaries separating the physical and metaphysical realms were less rigid than they might superficially appear. Within the broad-minded cultural context of the mid-nineteenth century, a number of schools of healing explored the intricate interconnections between the mind and the body and sought to unlock the therapeutic potential of untapped spiritual resources. For followers of hydropathy,

Thomsonianism, and homeopathy (to which would later be added osteopathy and chiropractic) the human mind was a microcosm of the divine and therefore a vast source of unrealized healing potential resided within every person. The power to cure disease and restore physical wellness, medical sectarians maintained, did not belong solely to formally trained practitioners of regular medicine.[6]

Following the disruption and carnage of the Civil War, a new metaphysical movement emerged in New England and grew throughout the United States, drawing its vitality from the nation's deep-seated yearning for solace and healing. Although at its root the metaphysical movement was an intellectual phenomenon, its adherents did not confine themselves solely to abstract and theoretical matters. As historian Catherine L. Albanese has observed, the movement "always spent its attentiveness on salving wounds and making people whole," forging new pathways to the improvement of humanity. "The New Age has nothing to fear, but everything to gain, from the rapidly advancing light of modern science," optimistically proclaimed the former- Methodist-turned-Swedenborgian minister Warren Felt Evans in 1864. "And that science will be the solid foundation on which the walls of the New Jerusalem will be built." In 1869 Evans published *The Mental Cure*, the first of several influential books he produced before his death in 1886. His works provided the foundation of one branch of the metaphysical movement, a loosely associated collection of seekers that most historical and literary scholars subsume under the umbrella of "New Thought." A second branch of the movement grew from Mary Baker Eddy's 1875 treatise *Science and Health* and became the legally incorporated entity known as of the First Church of Christ, Scientist. Although she shared many of his ideas about healing and the mind, Eddy viewed Evans and his numerous New Thought progeny as competitors and threats to her new church's legitimacy and to her own role as the earthly messenger of divine Truth. Maintaining a clear line of demarcation between the institutional religion of Christian Science and the ecumenical New Thought movement remained one of Eddy's lifelong endeavors.[7]

The intellectual lineages of both Warren Felt Evans and Mary Baker Eddy can be traced to a single person, Phineas Parkhurst Quimby. A clockmaker and autodidact Quimby, like many of his mid-nineteenth-century contemporaries, avidly explored the relationship between the physical and metaphysical realms. His ideas concerning the transmissions of bodily states between individuals represent one of many variations on a late eighteenth-century model established by the Viennese physician Franz Anton Mesmer.

Mesmer had posited that, when in proximity to each other, human beings became subject to mutually influencing forces, a phenomenon that paralleled the magnetism exhibited by certain minerals. He coined the term "animal magnetism" to refer to an unseen, fluid-like medium through which he postulated that human bodily states (hunger or sleepiness, for example) could be transferred from one person to another. Mesmer's ideas fall within a broader category of eighteenth-century "ether theories" that sought to explain how physical properties such as light, sound, and heat were transmitted across visibly empty space. Over time the label "mesmerism" came to be associated with any number of practices through which one person controlled the body of another using purely mental means. Mesmeric demonstrations would become a popular form of entertainment, shocking and often titillating middle-class audiences throughout Europe and the United States. Meanwhile, Mesmer himself developed a new therapeutic science predicated on his notion that he could use the power of his own animal magnetism to cure disease in others. He tested the efficacy of several techniques by which the healing transmissions might work, including physically touching the patient, gesturing toward and around the patient's body, and positioning magnets in various positions such as under the patient's feet, giving demonstrations of these variations before learned societies and lay audiences alike. While always controversial among both physicians and religious leaders, Mesmer's conceptual model of animal magnetism was nonetheless taken seriously and investigated rigorously by numerous medical researchers in both Europe and across the Atlantic.[8]

In 1838, in the small town of Belfast, Maine, Phineas Quimby attended a demonstration by a French mesmerist named Charles Poyen. Intrigued by what he witnessed, Quimby followed Poyen on the lyceum circuit throughout New England in order to study the precise nature of the conduits through which different bodily states might be transmitted. Soon Quimby began giving his own demonstrations of transference with the assistance of a partner named Lucius Burkmar. While in a trance state induced by Quimby, the young Burkmar diagnosed audience members' illnesses, seemingly able to see the presence of disease inside their bodies. Upon further investigation, however, Quimby became convinced that Burkmar's apparent gift was actually an exceptional interpersonal sensitivity that allowed him to discern what people *believed* to be true about their own physical states. From that premise Quimby deduced that it might be possible to rid people of their physical ailments by changing their thinking; the goal was to convince them they were in perfect health. Although he eventually rejected mesmerism per se (he even denounced Poyen, calling his original inspiration a "humbug"), throughout his life Quimby maintained a core belief that the root cause of human suffering lay in the power of suggestion. He developed a therapeutic practice predicated on the notion that individuals could be both sickened and cured strictly through mental transmissions. By the time of his death in 1866, Quimby's metaphysical therapy had attracted a substantial following of grateful patients who claimed he had relieved them of all manner of bodily ills that practitioners of regular medicine had failed to alleviate, or even made worse. One such patient was Mary Baker Eddy (then Mary Baker Patterson), a fellow New Englander who had spent much of her life tormented by sickness and invalidism. With her health at long last restored, Eddy became a devoted student of Quimby and his teachings, transcribing his dictated notes and developing a close intellectual relationship with the healer.[9]

Like many nineteenth-century Americans, Quimby held an expansive definition of what constituted science, developing his ideas within a loose intellectual framework with porous barriers that allowed him to cross rather easily between the physical and metaphysical realms. As historian Craig James Hazen notes, Quimby used the term "Science" in two distinct ways. The word sometimes referred to his own system of thought and healing practices, which he had arrived at through empirical observation and experimentation. But for Quimby "Science" also had a second, less prosaic meaning. He sometimes used the word to denote a cosmic and universal wisdom that, through the efforts of apostles like himself, would ultimately heal mankind at large. Throughout his writings Quimby used the term "Science" interchangeably with the word "God"; he also combined the concepts of divinity and knowledge within a single phrase, "Christian Science." Quimby's sacralization of science set a precedent that was subsequently emulated by numerous New Thought writers who also used the words "Science" and "God" synonymously. Significantly, in conflating the two realms Quimby neither denied the reality of the physical world nor denounced the validity of earthly observation and experimentation. To the contrary, as Hazen asserts, Quimby remained a "paradigmatic Baconian" throughout his life, maintaining "a spirited enthusiasm for natural science, propounding a scrupulous empiricism, and expressing an intense distrust of speculation." His suspicion of formal education and untutored reliance on inductive reasoning led Quimby to reject both regular medicine and organized religion because, he averred, neither could "stand the test of investigation." Ironically, in promoting empirical science as a source of absolute and universal authority, Quimby also unwittingly contributed to the growing dominance of regular over sectarian medicine that occurred in the half-century that followed his death.[10]

Although they did not occupy a central place in his writings (which remained unpublished in his own lifetime), children did appear in a few anecdotes Quimby used to illustrate the concept of transference. These stories also shed light on the techniques the healer employed in treating his patients. In one passage dating from the period 1860–1865, a mother sought Quimby's help for her mysteriously ailing five-year-old-son. When he queried the boy, however, the child simply responded that he often felt tired adding that, on occasion, his leg hurt after he had been playing. Quimby next asked the boy's mother to describe her own state of health, which she did by reciting an entire catalog of specific ailments: "A heavy feeling over the eyes, a numbness in the hands, weakness in the back, and pain going from the foot to the hip." Apparently in the habit of self-diagnosis, the woman told Quimby she was suffering from "spinal disease, trouble of the heart, and [she] was liable to have paralysis." After hearing her testimony Quimby noted that mother and son were, in fact, experiencing identical bodily symptoms but had simply articulated them very differently. "To her every sensation was the effect of some sort of disease," Quimby wrote of the mother, "yet every sensation she had the child had also, but had not attached names to them." From this observation the healer concluded that if she "had been as ignorant as the child of names, she would not have had the fear of those false ideas, and the child would have been well; for all its trouble came from its mother, and her trouble was the invention of the medical faculty." Thus in Quimby's analysis, the mother had turned her bodily experiences into specific disease states by attaching labels to them, and then transmitted the ailments to her young son.[11]

In another anecdote, Quimby described how he had determined the cause of a two-year-old patient's inability to walk properly, which a physician had previously diagnosed as a problem of the child's knee. Because the little boy was too young to answer questions, Quimby simply sat quietly with him until the healer himself "experienced a queer feeling in the hip and groin, but no bad feelings in the knee." He therefore concluded that the physician had been wrong and he relocated the source of the boy's disability. Quimby then redirected the mother's mental focus away from her son's knee and toward his hip. At Quimby's request she "put the child down and she could see that her will guided its motion." After witnessing this demonstration the mother came to understand the effect of her thoughts on her child's physical state. Next the healer successfully "changed the [mother's] mind so that the child walked much better." As these anecdotes from Quimby's writings illustrate, within his healing paradigm the transference property of animal magnetism applied to the bodies of children equally to those of adults. What is more, these passages suggest Quimby believed that the bodily states of both ease and disease moved with particular acuity when transmitted from mother to child.[12]

Mary Baker Eddy's teachings shared numerous key characteristics with those of her healer and mentor. She employed a distinctive lexicon (including the term "Christian Science" itself) that is also found in Quimby's unpublished writings and shared his foundational notions concerning the metaphysical transmissions of bodily states. But, despite the clear commonalities, Eddy engaged in a vigorous effort to distinguish Christian Science from Quimby's legacy (an effort sustained with equal ardor by a number of her contemporary and subsequent supporters). She laid out a defense of her doctrine's originality in the preface to *Science and Health* in which she claimed to have authored numerous works that were posthumously, and erroneously, attributed to Quimby. Eddy explained that, although at one time she had been naively persuaded by his ideas and methods, she now understood that in fact Quimby had been a "distinguished mesmerist" who had merely effected the appearance of curing her ailments. True and lasting healing came to Eddy only after "the revelation to me of the Principle of Christian Science" which she experienced some months after Quimby's death. Her recent revelations allowed her to see clearly that her predecessor's ideas and practices were self-evidently false because they had been arrived at using evidence from the material world. "When I conversed with [Quimby]," Eddy relayed to the readers of *Science and Health*, "he believed matter, sin, sickness, and death to be verities" rather than the mere illusions she knew them to be. After thus delegitimizing the work of Phineas Quimby, Eddy went on to denounce all practitioners of "mind cure" and its myriad derivations. "Various books on mental healing have been written in imitation of mine," she asserted in 1889, "but they are all more or less plagiaristic, and also incorrect."[13]

Nor were Eddy's efforts in staking out an exclusive claim to metaphysical healing limited to a war of words. She became embroiled in a number of legal actions as she struggled to maintain control over the new healing religion then growing rapidly both in Boston, which became its headquarters in 1882, and elsewhere in the United States. She sued a number of former students claiming they owed her royalties on fees they charged employing Christian Science healing techniques they had acquired under her tutelage. Several members of the new religion modified the tenets Eddy laid out in her treatise, publishing books and pamphlets of their own and attracting separate, and equally ardent, followings. In 1882 she successfully sued a former adherent and one-time personal friend Edward J. Arens for copyright infringement following Arens' publication of a pamphlet containing passages he had apparently lifted from *Science and Health*. Among the most notable insurgents was the enigmatic Josephine Curtis Woodbury, whose eccentric conduct and strident challenges to Eddy's leadership resulted in excommunication from the church; Woodbury then retaliated with a libel suit. Although the case was decided in Eddy's favor the legal triumph came only after her painful personal ordeal of the lengthy and widely publicized civil proceedings. In 1892, taking firm control over the precipitous and disorderly growth of the populist new healing religion, Eddy launched a major restructuring effort that limited executive power in the Christian Science church solely to herself and a small board of directors. The church's governance and practices were codified within a set of formal bylaws and services were modified to replace pastors with "readers" who recited pre-assigned passages from scripture and *Science and Health* without offering comments or interpretations. Befitting its by-now sizable following, the church relocated its headquarters from Lynn to Boston. As historian Beryl Satter has noted, the centralized and hierarchical nature of Christian Science provided a stable institutional structure that allowed the fledgling religion to survive its stormy formative years and, going forward, to far outpace a number of contemporary sects that were also centered around metaphysical healing practices. At the same time, however, Eddy's resolute rejection of modifications to her religious tenets addressing the nature of physical health and illness soon set Christian Science on a crash course with regular medicine and its practitioners.[14]

The healing paradigm promulgated by Mary Baker Eddy retained Phineas Quimby's notion of transference and the role of suggestion in causing and curing illness. Sufferers arrived at the Truth of perfect health when they came to understand that their belief in the existence of sickness was illusory, or Error. They reached the requisite awareness by reading the Bible and *Science and Health*. But Eddy acknowledged that such a profound change represented an extraordinarily difficult feat for ordinary people to accomplish, particularly for patients trapped within the torment and confusion of their false beliefs. The afflicted therefore had the option of employing healers who were trained and certified exclusively by the Christian Science church. The practitioner's role was to guide patients toward seeing the unreality of their physical distress, engaging them in a process of reasoning and argumentation. Significantly, the denial of material reality in Christian Science meant that church practitioners need not actually observe, speak to, touch, nor even come into the presence of the patient's physical body in order for this process to occur; healing could be effected telepathically via a method called "absent treatment." Further, Eddy taught that, just as Christian Science healed sickness by correcting Error in the mind of the sufferer, practitioners of methods other than Christian Science actually *caused* sickness by implanting Error when they acknowledged physical complaints and attached diagnostic labels to their patients' bodily experiences. "Common consent is contagious," she explained in an 1894 essay, "and it makes disease contagious." Regular medicine, with its preoccupation with naming diseases and tracing their etiologies, represented an especially pernicious source of human suffering. Thus for the most devout among Eddy's followers avoiding all contact with medical doctors was not merely a personal choice among a variety of available therapeutic regimes. Rather, eschewing medical care represented a religious imperative expressly put forth by their church's founder and codified within the church's laws.[15]

In a striking departure from her mentor's ideas, Eddy reframed the concept of animal magnetism in religious, indeed apocalyptic, terms. Like Franz Anton Mesmer, Phineas Quimby had explored what he believed to be a physical phenomenon, and as such it was amenable to observation and experimentation. By contrast, the founder of Christian Science used the term Malicious Animal Magnetism (which she often referred to as MAM) to mean an exceedingly dangerous metaphysical transmission capable of causing great harm, and even death. MAM was exploited by individuals who engaged in "malicious malpractice" by using the tenets of Christian Science, not to bring healing and solace to the suffering, but instead to exert control over the minds of others for their own evil purposes. Soon after her church was formally chartered, Eddy came to believe that a partner in her previous healing practice named Richard Kennedy was now engaged in malicious malpractice causing suffering to her personally as well as difficulties (legal and otherwise) for her fledgling church. In 1881 she added a forty-six-page chapter entitled "Demonology" to the third edition of *Science and Health* in which she detailed at length a convoluted narrative of crime and perfidy. She accused Kennedy, whom she referred to only as "the mesmerist," of numerous wicked acts including causing relapse and death in formerly cured patients and attempting to destroy Christian Science via slander and blackmail. "It is a law of metaphysics," Eddy asserted, "that the truth relating to health and being, when brought to bear upon mortal mind, acts favorably upon the body." But, she warned, "the mental mal-practitioner [like Kennedy] disregards the stern moral rules of metaphysics, and employs only that portion of our system which relates to the power of mind over body, and misuses that." MAM's mysterious and destructive power became even more apparent the following year when her third husband, Asa Gilbert Eddy, died unexpectedly, a tragedy she blamed on malicious mental transmissions sent by Edward J. Arens, the man she had sued for copyright infringement. Historian Catherine L. Albanese has observed that, despite her ardent commitment to the belief in God's perfection and loving power and the non-materiality of human sickness, Eddy's writings reflected a palpable sense of sin, evil, and human depravity as well as a "warfare model" of religion that reflected her New England childhood's immersion in a severe Calvinist theology. Until her death in 1910, Eddy and a close circle of trusted confidants fiercely protected the church and its healing practices from all competitors, both earthly and supernatural.[16]

In 1881 Eddy established the Massachusetts Metaphysical College to ensure that the church's healers would be trained strictly in accordance with Christian Science tenets. The Commonwealth of Massachusetts granted the new college a charter establishing it as an institution for the broad purpose of "teaching pathology, ontology, therapeutics, moral science, metaphysics, and their adaptation to the treatment of disease." Listing Dr. Mary Baker Eddy as its president, the college advertised itself as meeting "the demand of the age for something higher than physic or drugging to restore the race to hope and health." Initially at least, the physical location of the college was the living room of Eddy's home in Boston. Also in 1881, the church began a new publication, the *Christian Science Journal*, that featured stories of successful healings as Demonstrations of Truth, providing testimonials to the effectiveness of Christian Science therapeutics. True to her teachings, healers were strictly prohibited from utilizing any information or techniques derived from schools outside of the church's official doctrine. The college's Primary class, taught by Eddy herself or by one of her carefully chosen assistants, consisted of a twelve-lesson course, completion of which conferred the title S. C. B., or Bachelor of Christian Science. "If you have a thought higher than your patient," Eddy encouraged her Primary course students in 1889, "you will surely lift him with you." Upon completion of the Primary class students could proceed to a series of six lessons of advanced instruction, always taught by Eddy herself, which was called the Normal class. Those who completed both courses could then have their names listed in the *Christian Science Journal*, entitling them to advertise as certified church healers and to charge for their services. (A fee of one dollar per session was considered standard.) Other than full payment of all tuition (students were charged three hundred dollars for the Primary class and one hundred dollars for the Normal class; there was also a matriculation fee of five dollars) there were no qualifying examinations and, once granted, certification did not require any further education or training. After three years as an active healer, however, practitioners could use the title C. S. D., or Doctor of Christian Science. In the eight years it remained in operation, the Massachusetts Metaphysical College trained and certified approximately 800 healers, enabling the new practice to spread rapidly. Like a number of alternative and religious healing sects, Christian Science attracted a disproportionate number of women, most of whom remained locked out of regular medical education. In 1890, seventy-five percent of the church's practitioners were female; by 1910 that percentage had risen to eighty-nine.[17]

Relying solely on the metaphysical training they received at the Massachusetts Metaphysical College posed significant challenges for Christian Science practitioners called to attend cases involving sick or injured children. Eddy believed that children's bodies, like all human bodies, were manifestations of Error. But, because they lacked the requisite intellectual capacity to understand the unreality of their physical discomforts, children remained easily subject to transmitted fears, particularly from their overly anxious mothers. "If the child is exposed to contagion or infection," Eddy explained in *Science and Health*, "the mother is frightened and says 'my child will be sick.' The law of mortal mind and [a mother's] own fears govern her child more than the child's mind governs itself." The church's new bylaws prohibited official membership until the age of twelve, when it was assumed children became amenable to the process of reason and argumentation that constituted Christian Science healing. Thus in cases involving very young patients the practitioner's task was to bring parents to understand, not the illusion of their little one's sickness and suffering, but rather its authentic state of perfect health. The imperative to avoid transferring sickness through the medium of thought meant that Christian Science healers need not examine the body of the child, nor were they required to diagnose, or even to acknowledge physical symptoms; Christian Science practitioners did not typically provide palliative care.[18]

Outside of formal training at the Massachusetts Metaphysical College, Eddy devoted substantial sections of *Science and Health* to advising her followers on matters of child care. She dissuaded parents from attending too closely to their children's bodies because excessive attention only trained them to desire physical intimacy and comfort. "If parents create in their babes a desire for incessant amusement, to be always fed, rocked, tossed, or talked to, those parents should not, in after years, complain of their children's fretfulness or frivolity, which the parents themselves have occasioned," she admonished in her text. "Yielding one's thoughts to contemplate physical wants surely produces them." One year after Mary Putnam Jacobi's *Infant Diet* translated the latest pediatric perspectives on children's physical care to a popular audience, Eddy counseled her own followers along very different lines. "A single requirement, beyond what is necessary to meet the simplest needs of the base is harmful," she asserted. "Mind regulates the condition of the stomach, bowels, and food, the temperature of children and of men, and matter does not." Contrary to contemporary trends in regular medicine that advised close and continual scrutiny of children's bodies, Eddy warned that it was the constant seeking out of signs and symptoms of illness that actually posed a danger. Attending too closely would "convey mental images to children's budding thoughts, and often stamp them there, making it probable at any time that such ills may be reproduced in the very ailments feared." Parents should be equally wary of acknowledging their children's injuries lest they implant fear in young minds: "A mother runs to her little one, who has hurt her face by falling on the carpet, and says, moaning more childishly than her child, 'Mamma knows you are hurt.' The more successful method of treatment is to say: 'Oh, nonsense (no-sense material!). You're not hurt, so don't think you are'." Nor did children appear to have special needs for daily hygiene. Because the infant was naturally pure, Eddy explained, "the daily ablution of an infant is not more natural or necessary than to take a fish out of water and cover it with dirt, once a day, that it may thrive better in its natural element. Cleanliness is next to godliness, but washing should be only to keep the body clean, and this can be done with less than daily scrubbing the whole surface." Thus, in a clear and noteworthy departure from the late nineteenth-century's assignment of unprecedented importance to the physical care of children, Eddy's teaching implied that the best way for adults to deal with their children's needs was not to deal with them at all.[19]

Motherhood was a thorny subject in Mary Baker Eddy's lifetime, and it remained so among both her supporters and detractors long after her death in 1910. In 1844 Eddy was a young widow when she gave birth to her only biological child, George Glover. As a single mother bereft of resources she endured a peripatetic period living in poverty before returning to her parents' home in New Hampshire. But the next years were marred by difficulty. Eddy's health was very poor, her beloved mother passed away, and a man to whom she had become engaged to be married also died. Sympathetic accounts of Eddy's life often portray George as a difficult and fussy baby and an obstreperous little boy, the care of whom proved too much for his frail and financially distressed mother. Eddy either voluntarily or unwittingly (she used the phrase "my child was taken from me" in writing about this period) surrendered the six-year-old to the custody of her former maid, who took the boy to live in a New Hampshire village some forty miles away. She then married a dentist named Daniel Patterson who apparently wanted nothing to do with the boy and kept him away from the couple's home. In 1856, either with or without Eddy's cooperation (this point remains contested as well) George's foster parents took the now twelve-year-old child to live in Minnesota. Although Eddy divorced Patterson several years after he had deserted her for another woman, and she corresponded by mail with George, the boy was not in his mother's physical presence again for twenty-five years.[20]

The extended physical separation, Eddy's biographer Gillian Gill contends, lay at the root of Eddy's extensive bouts with ill health and invalidism during this difficult period in her life. Although she re-established contact with her grown son and his family, the relationship remained strained. In 1888, at the age of sixty-eight, Eddy legally adopted Ebenezer J. Foster, a forty-one-year-old man who had enrolled in her course at the Massachusetts Metaphysical College the previous year. That relationship, however, ended abruptly in personal turmoil. In 1907, Foster Eddy signed on with George Glover and several others as plaintiffs in a lawsuit charging that the eighty-five-year-old Eddy was no longer mentally competent to handle her extensive business affairs. Although the case against her was eventually withdrawn, her biographers agree that the ordeal took an immense personal toll on Eddy herself. Such unfortunate experiences with motherhood, of course, need not disqualify her as a source of authority on the physical care of children. After all, the two most important Enlightenment philosophers of childhood, John Locke and Jean Jacques Rousseau, were men who lacked direct personal experience in raising children. This much at least can be said: Eddy's own experience as a mother had been physically and emotionally fraught. Further, and perhaps more significantly, her time spent caring for a small child had taken place a full thirty years before she published the first edition of her treatise in 1875. Given these facts, it is not unreasonable to surmise that some mixture of psychological and chronological separation from her biological child, as well as her own challenging and painful associations with child-rearing, may be factors helping to explain Eddy's admonishments that parents maintain a psychological distance from the bodies of their children. Nor did new developments in medical science generally, and pediatrics specifically, have a place in the many subsequent revisions Eddy made to her church's foundational text. Nevertheless, reading *Science and Health* remained an essential element in the Christian Science healing process, including those who were caring for sick or injured children.[21]

Historian Beryl Satter has argued that Mary Baker Eddy was the most well-known and successful among a number of nineteenth-century female metaphysical leaders whose ideas were rooted in the denial of corporeal needs. These leaders associated the physical body and its urges, particularly sexual desire, with the primitive and destructive forces of men. According to Satter, Eddy's theology "hopefully predicted the end of both passion and marriage." Indeed, in *Science and Health* Eddy divorced procreation from physiology entirely; children seemingly materialize out of their parents' thoughts: "The so-called substance of bone," she asserted in *Science and Health*, "is formed first by the parent's mind, through self-division. Soon the child becomes a separate, individualized mortal mind, which takes possession of itself and its own thoughts of bones." Similarly, in an essay entitled "Wedlock" Eddy asserted that human procreation, along with birth and death, represented "subjective states of the erring mind." Maintaining the tenet of procreation by metaphysical means was not without risk, however. Eddy's biographer Gillian Gill explains that in 1890 Josephine Curtis Woodbury, the Christian Science healer who would be excommunicated nine years later, claimed to have immaculately conceived a son, apparently as a cover story for becoming pregnant while living apart from her husband. Woodbury stirred intense controversy by maintaining that *Science and Health*, as well as Eddy's teachings at the Massachusetts Metaphysical College, supported the notion of human procreation by spirit alone, an assertion that Eddy was forced to clarify in subsequent editions of *Science and Health*. "I discredit the belief that agamogenesis applies to the human species," she asserted. Even if Eddy conceded that the physical act of sex was necessary for conception, however, she stressed that it nevertheless should not take place during the course of the subsequent pregnancy.

"The Scientific morale of marriage is spiritual unity," Eddy wrote. "If the propagation of a higher human species is requisite to reach this goal, then its material conditions can only be permitted for the purpose of generating, the foetus must be kept mentally pure, and period of gestation have the sanctity of Virginity." Eddy's proscription on sex during pregnancy sought to protect the metaphysical fetus from the Error of the sensual maternal body in which it had been conceived and was developing.[22]

Given the vagaries of Eddy's views about human reproduction, it is perhaps not surprising that her church soon found itself embroiled in controversy over its practitioners' competence to attend cases of childbirth. In *Science and Health* Eddy instructed that "to attend properly the birth of the new child, you should so detach mortal thought from its material conceptions, that the birth will be natural and safe." In 1887 the Massachusetts Metaphysical College offered its first courses in metaphysical obstetrics, a series of six lessons at the cost of one hundred dollars, offered only to individuals who had successfully completed both the Primary and Normal courses. At this time Eddy began advertising herself as a "Professor of Obstetrics," a title that also appeared below her name in new editions of *Science and Health*. Initially the obstetrics course was taught by Eddy herself. "We have a certificate from the most celebrated and skillful Obstetrician and Surgeon in Massachusetts, stating our qualification to teach Obstetrics," a college flyer advertised. "And, what is better, our system prevents the suffering that has attended accouchement and with the great auxiliary of Mind, obviates the use of medicine." Several years previously Eddy had received a personal letter of certification in "accouchement" from a Dartmouth-trained physician named Rufus King Noyes, the president of an entity called the Bellevue Medical College that operated out of Lynn. In 1882, however, Noyes' institute lost its charter from the state of Massachusetts, apparently due to "irregular practices" that included mailing diplomas to people who had never actually attended the institute. In a strange twist, Noyes performed the autopsy on Asa Gilbert Eddy and concluded he had died of heart disease. When the widow insisted vehemently and publicly that he was wrong and her husband had been the victim of MAM, Noyes severed his connection to Eddy's college and prohibited any further use of his name in association with it. Another early associate was Charles J. Eastman who, despite having no medical training, had co-founded the Bellevue Medical College with Noyes and held the positions of professor of obstetrics and gynecology and dean there. Eastman, whom Eddy had known since childhood, was listed as a "consulting physician in surgery" at the Massachusetts Metaphysical College although it is unlikely that he gave any lectures. At the time the college opened he had already been indicted by a grand jury for performing an unspecified criminal operation (it is unclear whether it was an abortion), a charge he would face again in 1890 and then for a third time in 1893, when he was found guilty and sentenced to five years in prison following a patient's death. That year the Massachusetts legislature moved to prohibit institutions from granting degrees unless expressly authorized by the state to do so.[23]

Despite these problematic associations for Eddy's college she went forward with offering courses in metaphysical obstetrics and also gave lectures on human reproduction that were open to the public. The highly critical book published in 1909 by Willa Cather and Georgine Milmine charged that Eddy's teaching in the obstetrical course was "exceedingly informal and unsystematic" and dwelled excessively on the topic of MAM. These criticisms purportedly had been made by several students in the course, who also reported that they had been instructed to address medical complications such as premature labor and abnormal presentation by denying their material reality. *The Christian Science Journal*, by contrast, published glowing testimonials attesting to the value of metaphysical obstetrics. For example, a woman named Mrs. Ellen J. Fluno of Lexington described giving birth "entirely without pain" and attended only by her husband. Mrs. Fluno explained that she had previously taken a course from Eddy in which she learned that "mortal conception, birth, growth, and decay are all delusions, resulting from a finite sense of existence, which the truth of Being ignores." In any case, Eddy's foray into obstetrics was rather short-lived. In March 1888, a graduate of the Massachusetts Metaphysical College named Abby Corner was tried in Boston on the serious charge of felony manslaughter in the deaths of a mother and her stillborn infant. Compounding the tragedy was the fact that the victims were the healer's own daughter and granddaughter. The public response to Corner was hostile, particularly after the medical examiner ruled that the mother had hemorrhaged after giving birth and then bled to death over the course of three entire hours. The official insisted the mother would have survived under the care of "any midwife or nurse"—health care practitioners who regularly attended childbirth cases and whose training and experience was likely to include taking actions to stop hemorrhagic bleeding. Amid the controversy, Eddy not only distanced herself from Corner, but also joined in publicly denouncing her former pupil. In a letter sent to both the *Boston Globe* and the *Boston Herald*, Eddy explained that Corner had only completed one term of study at the Massachusetts Metaphysical College in 1886 rather than the requisite four, and her matriculation had occurred one year before the specialized obstetrical course had been initiated. Corner, therefore, "was not fitted at this institute for an accoucheur." Going further, Eddy admonished that "recreant practitioners in any school of medicine are a disgrace to it." Of course, at the time childbirth remained a hazardous undertaking regardless of whether physicians, nurses, midwives, or Christian Science healers were in attendance. No doubt with some recognition of that reality, the jury acquitted Corner of the criminal charge.[24]

The tragic Corner case raised serious doubts about the adequacy of the obstetrical training provided at the Massachusetts Metaphysical College and also brought both unprecedented awareness of, and scrutiny toward, practitioners of the rapidly growing vocation of Christian Science healing. The late nineteenth century saw a fierce battle among sectarian health care practitioners over control of the medical marketplace, a struggle led aggressively by regular physicians represented by the American Medical Association. In the midst of the battle over professional turf, however, a fundamental question remained to be answered: Could a therapeutic paradigm that denied the physical reality of both maternal and fetal bodies adequately prepare Christian Scientists to assist in childbirth cases, particularly when complications arose? Eddy's followers divided over the answer. For a number of years following the Corner controversy Christian Science healers continued attending births, and the church's publications regularly printed testimonials from mothers extolling their positive experiences, particularly the absence of fear and pain. Nevertheless, the terrible circumstances of the Corner case and its damage to the reputation of Christian Science prompted some practitioners to advocate a compromise in which they would combine their metaphysical training with either allopathic or homeopathic medical education. Mixing Christian Science with materia medica, however, remained specifically forbidden in the church's bylaws; violators risked not only decertification as healers but expulsion from church membership as well. The impasse over metaphysical obstetrics resulted in the exit of one-third of the church's practitioners in Boston, a conflict that served to prolong public scrutiny of Christian Science healing.[25]

Although Eddy repeatedly asserted that the controversy was the work of MAM, she also took practical steps to shield the Massachusetts Metaphysical College from future legal liabilities. In March 1888, the same month the Corner incident took place, a notice appeared in the *Christian Science Journal* announcing that Eddy herself would cease teaching the Normal course.

The following November the *Boston Herald* published a press release from unsigned "members of the Christian Science Church" attempting to clarify the college's training of health care practitioners and, hopefully, put an end to the criticism that the college was grossly negligent in claiming to train students in the practice of obstetrics:

> This statement that the Massachusetts Metaphysical College is a medical college is erroneous. It does not purport in any sense to be a medical college, but a college which teaches exclusively metaphysical and spiritual healing. We regard this as a very important matter, in view of the fact that repeated attempts have been made to place Christian Scientists before the public in the attitude of medical practitioners.

The following year the college was reorganized as an auxiliary of the church, identifying it more directly as a religious rather than a medical institution. Nevertheless, it continued operations under a new director of teaching, Erastus M. Bates. Bates, in turn, employed Eddy's newly adopted son Ebenezer J. Foster Eddy to teach an obstetrics course. A graduate of Hahnemann Medical College in Philadelphia, Foster Eddy had a medical license and had practiced as a homeopathic physician in Vermont before eschewing his training and entering the Massachusetts Metaphysical College. "I have tried this system of treatment in obstetrics with vastly improved results over the old way," he declared in a speech before the Vermont Homeopathic Medical Society. "Physicians, not in the line of Christian Science, can testify their surprise at witnessing the labor at childbed rendered painless by the aid of Christian Scientists, which, all must admit, is a new experience." Eddy and Foster Eddy co-taught the obstetrics course, with Foster Eddy leading courses in anatomy and physiology and Eddy providing lessons in metaphysics.[26]

By the end of the nineteenth century, the church took further steps to shore up the legitimacy of its healing practices and sought to curb the activities of its competitors. Eddy began requiring one member of the church's Board of Education to have a Massachusetts medical license, presumably to advise on the increasingly stringent restrictions on the practice of medicine in the state. Between 1899 and 1901 the church employed Alfred E. Baker, who was both a regular medical doctor and a Christian Scientist, to teach some lessons in metaphysical obstetrics. As historian Rennie B. Schoepflin observed, Baker's lecture notes clearly demonstrate that deep pitfalls remained in the teaching and practice of metaphysical childbirth. Baker instructed birth attendants to remain mentally detached from the physical needs of both mother and baby throughout the birthing process, a position that appears problematic at best and professionally negligent at worst. The not-uncommon risks of puerperal fever and ruptured peritoneum were nonexistent. Practitioners must guard against implanting Error in newborns' consciousness by looking too closely at them; they must not assess babies' physical appearance, even to identify their sex, and they must not touch the umbilical cord. Nor should attendants worry if a baby fails to nurse since, as Baker enigmatically noted, there could be "no loss to [a] child because of [a] lack of nutrition." At the turn of the twentieth century, such instruction seemed startlingly out of touch with the increasingly prevalent belief that the body of the child deserved the highest level of care and concern. Also at this time, Christian Science healers in a number of states faced legal prosecution for committing infractions such as failing to report communicable diseases to local public health officials and practicing medicine in violation of newly strengthened medical licensing requirements. In 1902, just as the first trials of Christian Scientist *parents* who had failed to provide medical assistance to their dying children hit the headlines, the *Christian Science Journal* abruptly and enigmatically announced that "Obstetrics is not [Christian] Science, and will not be taught." Eddy's decision to simply excommunicate childbirth from her teachings resolved the seemingly intractable risks to the institutional church inherent in the venture of metaphysical obstetrics. But, for her devout followers faced with the profound dilemma of providing care to their sick and injured children, the resolution of the problem could not be so perfunctory.[27]

## NOTES

1. Mary Baker G. Eddy, *Science and Health with Key to the Scriptures*. Fortieth edition (Boston: Mary Baker G. Eddy, 1889), 412.
2. Eddy, *Science and Health* (1889), 12; Rodney Stark, "The Rise and Fall of Christian Science," *Journal of Contemporary Religion*, Volume 13, Number 2 (1998): 189–214; Deborah Madden, *A Cheap, Safe, and Natural Medicine": Religion, Medicine, and Culture in John Wesley's Primitive Physic* (Rodopi Press, 2007); Walter I. Wardell, "Christian Science Healing," *Journal for the Scientific Study of Religion*, Volume 4, Number 2 (Spring 1965): 171–181; and Margaret M. Poloma, "A Comparison of Christian Science and Mainline Christian Healing Ideologies and Practices," *Review of Religious Research*, Volume 32, Number 4 (June 1991): 337–350.

3. Eddy, *Science and Health* (1889), 155; Stephen Gottschalk, *Rolling Away the Stone: Mary Baker Eddy's Challenge to Materialism* (Bloomington: Indiana University Press, 2006), 6.

4. Eddy, *Science and Health* (1889), 530, 335.

5. Eddy, *Science and Health* (1889), 12, 320; Norman Gevitz, "Christian Science Healing and the Health Care of Children," *Perspectives in Biology and Medicine*, Volume 34, Number 3 (Spring 1991): 421–438.

6. On sectarian medicine in the nineteenth century see: Norman Gevitz, editor, *Other Healers: Unorthodox Medicine in America* (Johns Hopkins University Press, 1988); Robert C. Fuller, *Alternative Medicine and American Religious Life* (New York: Oxford University Press, 1989); James C. Whorton, *Nature Cures: The History of Alternative Medicine in America* (Oxford University Press, 2002); and Martha M. Libster, *Herbal Diplomats* (Neenah, WI: Golden Apple Publications, 2004).

7. Peter Manseau, *The Apparitionists* (Boston: Houghton Mifflin 2017), 6–7; Catherine L. Albanese, *A Republic of Mind and Spirit: A Cultural History of American Metaphysical Religion* (Yale University Press, 2007), 15; and Warren Felt Evans, *The New Age and Its Messenger* (Boston: T.H. Carter and Company, 1864), 107. For older scholarly interpretations of the metaphysical movement see also J. Stillson Judah, *The History and Philosophy of Metaphysical Movements in America* (Westminster Press, 1967); Charles S. Braden, *Spirits in Rebellion: The Rise and Development of New Thought* (University Park, TX: Southern Methodist University Press, 1963).

8. Allison Winter, *Mesmerized: Powers of Mind in Victorian Britain* (Chicago: University of Chicago Press, 1998), 1–13; Adam Crabtree, *From Mesmer to Freud: Magnetic Sleep and the Roots of Psychological Healing* (New Haven: Yale University Press, 1993), 115–137; and Robert Darnton, *Mesmerism and the End of the Enlightenment in France*. Revised edition (Cambridge, MA: Harvard University Press, 1986), 46–81.

9. Albanese, *A Republic of Mind and Spirit*, 283–300; Craig James Hazen, *The Village Enlightenment in America: Popular Religion and Science in the Nineteenth Century* (Urbana: University of Illinois Press, 2000), 113–146; and Beryl Satter, *Each Mind a Kingdom: American Women, Sexual Purity, and the New Thought Movement, 1875–1920* (University of California Press, 1999), 59–64.

10. Hazen, *The Village Enlightenment in America*, 124–130. Although he provides his readers with a lucid analysis, Hazen also notes that Quimby's writings were neither consistently methodical nor completely coherent.

11. Phineas Parkhurst Quimby, "The Effect of Mind Upon Mind." In Horatio W. Dresser, editor, *The Quimby Manuscripts* (New York: The Julian Press, 1961), 257–260.

12. Quimby, "The Treatment of a Child." In Horatio W. Dresser, editor, *The Quimby Manuscripts* (New York: The Julian Press, 1961), 308–309.

13. Eddy, *Science and Health* (1889), 5–10. The nature and extent of Eddy's intellectual debt to Quimby is a topic with a long and contentious history. In 1909 Willa Cather and Georgine Milmine published a damning exposé, *The Life of Mary Baker G. Eddy and the History of Christian Science* (Doubleday, Page and Company). A more recent account by the writer, editor, and former church member Caroline Fraser is also extremely critical of Eddy: *God's Perfect Child: Living and Dying in the Christian Science Church* (New York: Henry Holt 1999). A comprehensive biography of Eddy was authored by Robert Peel, a Christian Scientist and church official, and published in three volumes: *Mary Baker Eddy: The Years of Discovery* (New York: Holt, Rinehart and Winston, 1966); *Mary Baker Eddy: The Years of Trial* (Holt, Rinehart and Winston, 1971); and *Mary Baker Eddy, The Years of Authority* (Holt, Rinehart and Winston, 1977). Treatments of Eddy that are both scholarly and sympathetic include Gottschalk, *Rolling Away the Stone*; Gillian Gill, *Mary Baker Eddy* (New York: Perseus Books, 1998); and Claire Hoertz Badaracco, *Prescribing Faith: Medicine, Media, and Religion in American Culture* (Waco, TX: Baylor University Press, 2007).

14. Beryl Satter, *Each Mind a Kingdom: American Women, Sexual Purity, and the New Thought Movement, 1875–1920* (Berkeley: University of California Press, 1999), 1–10; Stephen Gottschalk, *Rolling Away the Stone*, 90–91; and Albanese, *A Republic of Mind and Spirit*, 315–322.

15. Mary Baker Eddy, "Contagion." In *Miscellaneous Writings 1883–1896* (Boston: Trustees under the will of Mary Baker G. Eddy, 1924), 228–229.

16. Mary B. Glover Eddy, *Science and Health*, Volume II. Third edition revised (Lynn, MA: Dr. Asa G. Eddy, 1881), 40; Albanese, *A Republic of Mind and Spirit*, 290–291. For a discussion of Eddy's protracted feuds with Richard Kennedy and Edward J. Arens see Gottschalk, *Rolling Away the Stone*, 90–91, 266–267, 381.

17. Massachusetts Metaphysical College Records, Box #155, Folder SF, "Charter, Copy, Correspondence" and Box #155, Folder HF, "Circulars and Curriculum Notes." The Mary Baker Eddy Library, Boston, Massachusetts. Although Eddy claimed to have taught 4000 students at the College, records of the Mary Baker Eddy Library put the documented number at 800. See Michael R. Davis, "'Loving Care and Counsel': Mary Baker Eddy's Letters of Advice to Healers," *The Mary Baker Eddy Library for the Betterment of Humanity*, Volume 4, Number 3 (2005): 10–15. The degrees granted by the Massachusetts Medical College are explained in "Degrees from the Massachusetts Metaphysical College," *Christian Science Journal*, Volume V, Number 7 (October 1887): 378. For a discussion of the training and curriculum at the college see Rennie B. Schoepflin, *Christian Science on Trial: Religious Healing in America* (Baltimore: Johns Hopkins University Press, 2003), 33–53.

18. Eddy, *Science and Health* (1889), 334; Gill, *Mary Baker Eddy*, 414–417. On the significance of women in nineteenth-century sectarian medicine see Naomi Rogers, "Women and Sectarian Medicine." In Rima D. Apple,

editor, *Women, Health, and Medicine in America: A Historical Handbook* (Rutgers University Press, 1992); Jane B. Donegan, *"Hydropathic Highway to Health": Women and Water-Cure in Antebellum America* (New York: Greenwood Press, 1986).

19. Mary Baker Glover, *Science and Health with Key to the Scriptures* (Boston: Christian Scientist Publishing Company, 1875), 319–320; Eddy, *Science and Health* (1889), 335–336.

20. Gottschalk, *Rolling Away the Stone*, 20–42, 155–163. Eddy published a memoir, *Retrospection and Introspection*, that rather obliquely references her separation from George (Boston: Trustees of the First Church of Christ, Scientist, 1891).

21. Gill, *Mary Baker Eddy*, 68–115.

22. Satter, *Each Mind a Kingdom*, 73–79; Eddy, *Science and Health* (1893), 271, 421; Mary Baker Eddy, *Miscellaneous Writings 1883–1896* (Boston: Trustees of the First Church of Christ, Scientist, 1893), 286; Gill, *Mary Baker Eddy*, 418–449; and Mary Baker Eddy, *Science and Health with Key to the Scriptures* (Boston: Trustees of the First Church of Christ, Scientist, 1906), 68.

23. Eddy, *Science and Health* (1893), 447; Records of the Massachusetts Metaphysical College, Box #155, Folder SF, "Charter, Copy, Correspondence"; Box #156, Folder "Charles J. Eastman," Folder "Jane C. Howard Material," Folder "Correspondence 1890–1911." The Mary Baker Eddy Library, Boston, Massachusetts; "A Bogus Medical College—The Massachusetts Bellevue," *Annual Report of the Illinois State Board of Health 1880* (Springfield: H.W. Rocker, 1881): 13–18; Willa Cather and Georgine Milmine, *The Life of Mary Baker G. Eddy and the History of Christian Science* (New York: Doubleday Page and Company, 1909; Reprinted by the University of Nebraska Press, 1993), 289.

24. Cather and Milmine, *The Life of Mary Baker G. Eddy*, 352–336; Mrs. Ella V. Fluno, "Obstetrics," *The Christian Science Journal*, Volume V, Number 8 (November 1887): 395. Abby Corner's name appears on a list of graduates of the Massachusetts Medical College. Records of the Massachusetts Metaphysical College, Box #156, Folder "1886 Curriculum." The Mary Baker Eddy Library, Boston, Massachusetts.

25. Gill, *Mary Baker Eddy*, 347–348; Schoepflin, *Christian Science on Trial*, 95–101.

26. E. J. Foster, "Homeopathic Materia Medica the Material Stepping-Stone to Christian Science Mind-Cure," *The Christian Science Journal*, Volume VI, Number 7 (October 1888): 325–330; "Massachusetts Metaphysical College," *The Christian Science Journal*, Volume VI, Number 7 (October 1888): 375.

27. Schoepflin, *Christian Science on Trial*, 106, 246, notes 60, 61.

# CHAPTER 5

# The Infected Child

In the next tube rests a yellowish white germ of flimsy texture and almost transparent. Three words full of meaning to those who have sat by the bedside of a dying child mark it as one of the greatest enemies of the human race: *bacillus Corynebacterium diphtheriae.*

Beginning in the 1880s, the new science of bacteriology engendered a great deal of optimism that before long a number of deadly diseases would be conquered. The German physician Robert Koch built upon the germ theory pioneered by the French microbiologist Louis Pasteur to identify the specific bacteria that caused anthrax, tuberculosis, and cholera. The American public's fascination with the new laboratory science in Europe is reflected in a *Chicago Daily Tribune* article sporting the jarring headline, "Bottled Up Death." The reporter extolled the virtues of a bacteriology exhibit then on display at the World's Columbian Exposition—a five-month-long event mounted on a colossal scale that was itself intended as a tribute to western progress. At the exhibit, the *Tribune* writer explained, members of the public could view the bacillus that caused diphtheria, a contagious and much-dreaded disease that took the lives of thousands of children each year. Lest such a sight cause undue anxiety, the *Tribune* reassured its readers that "German professors" were hard at work finding cures for diphtheria as well as for a panoply of other contagious diseases, ushering

© The Author(s) 2019
L. Curry, *Religion, Law, and the Medical Neglect
of Children in the United States, 1870–2000,*
Palgrave Studies in the History of Childhood,
https://doi.org/10.1007/978-3-030-24689-1_5

in nothing less than a new scientific age when "the terrors of cholera and other plagues will be things of the past." In 1893, as throngs of fair-goers in Chicago peered at a colony of *Corynebacterium diphtheriae* growing in a test tube made of glass, officials in New York City's Public Health Department issued a new directive that required laboratory diagnoses to be carried out in all suspected cases of diphtheria.[1]

Children were often posited as the special beneficiaries of the new laboratory-based medicine. At the close of the nineteenth century, children under the age of five accounted for a staggering proportion of annual deaths; one New York official put the ratio as high as one-third for that city. Most of these untimely deaths resulted from infectious ailments falling within two general categories: respiratory and diarrheal diseases. As the *Chicago Daily Tribune* enthusiastically noted, the possibility of an effective new weapon to combat diphtheria was among the most promising of developments coming from bacteriology. Regular physicians were very well acquainted with the disease and the frightening "pseudomembrane" associated with its progress in the body of the sufferer, a product of toxic discharges that grew to cover patients' throats and nasal passages. Multiple cases within the same household were common, and it appeared that children could contract the ailment more than once. In a best-selling personal memoir recounting his early years in medical practice, the Kansas physician Arthur E. Hertzler vividly recalled his young diphtheria patients' high fevers, rapid pulse rates, bleeding nasal passages, and distinctly blue faces as they threw back their heads and shoulders in the struggle to breathe. Once witnessed, Hertzler's description made clear, a fatal case of diphtheria was impossible to forget. In 1880, Abraham Jacobi's *Treatise on Diphtheria* cataloged for a readership of medical doctors an extensive set of possible bodily symptoms, describing in detail variations in the location, appearance, and odor of the pseudomembrane as the disease took its course.[2]

And yet, prior to the 1890s, the scientific medical community remained quite divided over the most effective ways to go about identifying, classifying, and battling this childhood scourge. Diphtheria was an especially wily adversary because, in its early stages, it was difficult to distinguish from other serious respiratory ailments that affected the mucous membranes such as croup and scarlet fever. The disease presented differently in individual cases, seeming to take either milder or more virulent forms. A sufferer's chances of asphyxiation were affected by the specific area covered by the pseudomembrane. A further, and considerable, complication was that diphtheria appeared to kill its victims in more than one way. Besides suffocation, fatal damage to the nervous system and kidneys, as well as a sudden paralysis of the heart muscle, sometimes occurred in patients—even after the pseudomembrane had cleared or was expelled and the child appeared to be recovering. Given its widely variable presentation, then, medical researchers debated whether "diphtheria" actually constituted a single childhood ailment or several. As a result, physicians and parents who must rely exclusively on observing a sick child's bodily symptoms faced considerable difficulties in assessing the risk the disease posed to a child's life. Parents needed to make critical and timely decisions about if, and when, they would seek the services of a physician to aid their stricken child.[3]

Uncertainties over diphtheria's causes and symptoms led to disagreements over the best way to treat infected patients. In his 1880 treatise Abraham Jacobi considered a long list of therapies intended to dissolve the pseudomembrane including washes, atomized mists, and inhaled steams to which were added a variety of substances ranging in severity from lime water to carbolic acid. While mild substances worked too slowly (if at all), harsh ones risked severely damaging surrounding tissue permanently, and perhaps even fatally. But, if washes were unsatisfactory, Jacobi also warned physicians against attempting to expel the pseudomembrane by administering emetics in order to induce vomiting. He also rejected the use of surgical or mechanical instruments because, in addition to posing an unacceptable risk of harming young patients, the pseudomembrane invariably grew back quickly anyway, negating even the slight chance that such a dangerous procedure would succeed. Surveying the range of unsatisfactory options, Jacobi was only slightly more impressed with tracheotomy, a centuries-old procedure in which the physician opened the trachea via a surgical incision so that patients suffering from laryngeal stenosis (constriction of the airway) could breathe. In 1826 the French physician Pierre Bretonneau, who was the first to use the word *diphtherité* (membrane) to identify the disease, began to perform tracheotomies in an attempt to aid his asphyxiating patients. But the surgery posed considerable risks of its own; tracheotomies often killed patients outright or else introduced infection from other bacteria which destroyed their already weakened bodies. Further, the tracheal opening commonly failed to stay clear enough to allow adequate breathing to continue only hours after the dangerous procedure had been performed. The fact that tracheotomy was generally regarded as an extreme measure to be used only as a last resort when patients were already asphyxiating undoubtedly played a role in the operation's frustratingly low rate of success. Writing in 1880, Jacobi described his own attempts to use tracheotomy in diphtheria cases as unqualified failures.[4]

Five years after Jacobi's *Treatise on Diphtheria* appeared in print Joseph O'Dwyer, a young physician with the New York Foundling Asylum, derived an intubation procedure that could be used in place of high-risk tracheotomies. O'Dwyer's intubation method represented a significant improvement because it was fast and required no anesthetic. Rather than a surgical incision, O'Dwyer's procedure utilized specialized tubes, originally made of brass and later of rubber, which the physician inserted into the larynx to create an alternative airway. The tubes were produced in several different sizes to fit patients from infancy to adolescence. But intubation was not without risks and appeared to be a rather harrowing experience itself, as described by O'Dwyer himself in an 1889 publication entitled *Intubation in Croup and Other Acute and Chronic Forms of Stenosis of the Larynx*. An illustration in the text depicted a nurse seated on a chair holding a small child on her lap; a physician's assistant stood behind the nurse and the child while the physician or "operator" stood in front of the trio. O'Dwyer noted that seeking the assistance of others was always necessary because "children seldom remain long in one position when suffering severely from want of breath." The assistant held the child's head firmly and slightly backward as the operator first inserted a "Denhart gag" to prop open the child's mouth; this was to be followed as quickly as possible by operator inserting the tube using an instrument called the "introducer." Because this procedure required greater manual dexterity than the average non-surgeon practitioner was likely to have acquired, O'Dwyer advised against attempting it on live (and presumably struggling) patients without first practicing on cadavers. "The operator has so many things to think of," he warned, "and so many movements to make with both hands, all in a few seconds, that unless [the physician has] sufficient practice to make some of these movements to a certain extent automatic, he cannot operate with safety to his patient or credit to himself." Despite its clear risks and anxiety-inducing implementation, intubation offered significant hope in what were otherwise very dismal circumstances. As historian Anne Hardy observed, O'Dwyer's method allowed non-surgeons who were adequately trained to employ the life-saving procedure, boosting the visibility and prestige of the new medical specialty of pediatrics. The new field's leaders wagered it was far better to offer "something rather than nothing" to anxious parents as they helplessly witnessed their child's struggle to breathe. Abraham Jacobi overcame his own initial skepticism to become an enthusiastic endorser of O'Dwyer's method and within ten years of its introduction intubation replaced tracheotomy as the most commonly used intervention for diphtheria cases in the United States.[5]

Meanwhile, diphtheria raged on. Although it was an endemic rather than an epidemic disease in the United States, cases spiked periodically, and inexplicably, in particular geographic locations. New York City, the home of Abraham and Mary Putnam Jacobi, was no exception. In June 1883, the Jacobis' seven-year-old son Ernst died after contracting diphtheria; his three-year-old sister also came down with the disease but fortunately she survived. That two of the most prominent American physicians of the late nineteenth century were not themselves spared from personal tragedy served as a poignant reminder that diphtheria remained a deadly, and in many ways a mysterious, ailment. To many in the regular medical community, it may have seemed inconceivable that parents possessing such a wealth of medical knowledge and experience nevertheless remained helpless to protect their own children from diphtheria's scourge. Somehow, these physicians had overlooked the danger that lurked within their household. As parents the Jacobis were devastated. Mary Jacobi wrote a friend describing her feelings of "self-contempt" as well as her certainty that "the whole world" now judged her to be a failure. Interestingly, the Jacobis directed their suspicions about the source of contagion, not on the possible role played by their own exposure to diphtheria through their work, but rather on the family's German immigrant nurse. Upon being questioned the nurse admitted that she had, in fact, experienced bouts of sore throat just prior to the onset of each child's illness but had kept her condition hidden from her employers, perhaps fearing they would send her away. The Jacobis shipped the nurse back to Germany.[6]

Following Ernst's death Abraham Jacobi focused his prodigious professional attention to the enduring mystery of diphtheria contagion. He published a provocative article in the *New York Medical Journal* entitled "Diphtheria Spread by Adults" that historian Evelynn Maxine Hammond has characterized as nothing less than a "polemic about the cause and transmission of diphtheria." Jacobi challenged the prevailing medical view in the United States that the locus of infection lay remotely in the environment (particularly environments inhabited by the poor) where it was spontaneously generated by noxious odors, filth, or dampness. He made the discomforting argument that the source more likely lurked much closer to the ailing child itself. Because some cases appeared relatively mild, diphtheria was often misdiagnosed by sufferers and physicians alike as any one of a number of more benign illnesses that presented with similar symptoms. As a result, people infected with diphtheria and experiencing only mild sore throat, or perhaps no symptoms at all, might come into close contact with children and unknowingly transmit the disease. Drawing upon his own vast clinical experience, Jacobi cited several cases that appeared to bolster his argument that diphtheria was spread by close human contact. His most notable example involved a brother and sister who, although seemingly healthy, nevertheless contracted diphtheria, which the little girl survived but her older brother did not. Only subsequently did the parents learn that their "old, trusted, and trustworthy" nurse had concealed her own attacks of a sore throat from her employers. Jacobi used this thinly disguised account of his own personal tragedy to urge physicians to "look for the cause of every case of diphtheria in the nares and throats" of the adults who had come into close contact with a stricken child. The prominent pediatrician concluded the article by wistfully noting that the absolute necessity of conducting such careful surveillance had only "dawned on me too late."[7]

If Jacobi's suspicion about the source of contagion pointed in a generally bacteriological direction, his theory nevertheless fell short of identifying any single culprit. But the article appeared at a critical moment, halfway through a decade in which the new laboratory science linked anthrax, cholera, and tuberculosis to the presence of specific bacteria. Although a great deal of attention was also being given to the scientific study of diphtheria, determining even basic scientific facts about the disease proved challenging. Laboratory specimens taken from young patients suffering from sore throats and inflamed mucous membranes invariably contained several different strains of bacteria, including the streptococcus bacillus, an equally virulent source of much serious childhood illness and death. Then in 1884, the same year that Jacobi's challenge to the medical community appeared in the *New York Medical Journal*, the Swiss pathologist Edwin Klebs and the German bacteriologist Freidrich Loeffler narrowed the list of suspects by identifying the diphtheria bacillus. While the work of Klebs and Loeffler represents a seminal event in the history of bacteriology, historical scholarship has demonstrated that it only marked the beginning of a complex transition in which the disease known as diphtheria came to be defined by the presence of *Corynebacterium diphtheriae* rather than by a set of physical symptoms exhibited in the body. Significantly, a definitive diagnosis of "true" diphtheria could be made only through laboratory analysis rather than solely by scrutinizing its manifestation in the body of the child.

Many in the regular medical community balked at ceding their professional prerogative to diagnose and treat illness to pathology laboratories, particularly since most practicing physicians lacked access to these new sites of medical authority. Thus a gap between the laboratory and the sick child's bedside remained unbridged.[8]

In 1892, William Hallock Park devised a simple procedure in which he swabbed patients' pseudomembranes and introduced the sample into a glass tube that had been previously prepared with blood serum. Visible colonies of bacteria quickly grew in the tubes, which could then be stained and examined under a microscope for definitive identification. Park had trained in New York with T. Mitchell Prudden, one of a handful of Americans who in the 1880s brought the new science of bacteriology to the United States from Europe. The following year Hermann M. Biggs of the New York City Department of Health announced a plan to distribute materials to doctors for use in collecting specimens, which they could then send to the city's newly established pathology laboratory for analysis. Within twenty-four hours they could receive a definitive diagnosis of diphtheria, information that allowed them to better monitor patients lest a dramatic intervention such as intubation become necessary to save a life. In addition, a positive identification of the diphtheria bacillus enabled actions to be taken to stop the disease from spreading to other children. Writing as the new director of the health department's Division of Pathology, Bacteriology, and Disinfection, Park provided a detailed description of his system in the *New York Medical Record* in which he instructed physicians in preparing the test tubes and swabbing the pseudomembrane. In addition to its benefits for the diphtheria sufferer, Park stressed the value of early and accurate diagnosis for preventing diphtheria's spread. "Care for the public health," he asserted, "requires that every case of possible diphtheria be properly isolated and treated as diphtheria until all doubt is removed." Park concluded that in ambiguous or doubtful cases it was nothing less than "the duty of physicians to obtain a diagnosis by the use of cultures" rather than relying solely on their own powers of observation. Following New York City's lead, by 1900 public health departments in many major American cities had established diagnostic facilities. The medical gaze, meticulously fixed on the body of the child for over a century, had now expanded its focus to take in microscopic information imparted by the pathology laboratory.[9]

Weighing in on these new developments, leading pediatricians stressed the complementary nature of laboratory and clinical evidence in diagnosing diphtheria. "While bacteriological diagnosis is, on the whole, more exact,"

Luther Emmett Holt wrote in 1897, "it should not be depended upon to the exclusion of clinical diagnosis. The prevailing tendency to disregard the clinical evidence and rely wholly upon bacteriology is greatly to be deprecated." In his textbook *The Diseases of Infancy and Childhood*, Holt apprised his physician readership of the new, bacteriologically based, definition of diphtheria: "In the following pages the term *diphtheria* will be limited to those cases in which the Klebs-Loeffler bacillus is present, the others being grouped under the head of false or *pseudo-diphtheria*. Diphtheria may then be defined as an acute, specific, communicable disease due to the bacillus of Klebs and Loeffler." Plates reproduced from Park's published work contrasted diphtheria and streptococcus bacteria as they appeared under a microscope. After establishing the bacteriological foundation for the reader, Holt went on to discuss diphtheria's appearance in the body of the child: "It is usually characterized by the formation of a false membrane upon certain mucous membranes, especially those of the tonsils, pharynx, nose, or larynx." Finally, the influential pediatrician warned about the range of variation that doctors were likely may see among diphtheria cases: "Like other pathogenic organisms, however, this germ acts with varying forms of intensity, and may cause inflammation of all degrees of severity, from a mild catarrhal angina to the most serious membrane inflammation; but to all alike the term diphtheria should be applied." In the ensuing pages Holt provided a lengthy discussion of how the variations in diphtheria's virulence might present in differing observable symptoms, enabling informed doctors to diagnose and assess the severity of a case without, or perhaps prior to, obtaining a definitive bacteriological analysis. In the most dangerous cases, he cautioned, the onset of the disease was both sudden and severe and thus there was no valid reason to wait for laboratory confirmation before regarding a suspicious case to be diphtheria and taking appropriate measures. The pseudomembrane appeared and grew very rapidly and in fact was capable of extending over the throat and nasal passages within a mere twenty-four hours; Holt's text provided three color plates for doctors to use as a visual aid in recognizing danger. An attending physician might also observe bloody discharges emanating from a patient's nose and throat. In the worst cases a generalized constitutional failing appeared within two to five days. Warning signs that toxins had spread more generally throughout the body could be seen in "extreme muscular weakness and prostration, by a feeble, rapid pulse, and a mental state of apathy or stupor, sometimes alternating with great restlessness." While not all diphtheria cases advanced to this dire state, Holt cautioned that "so many possibilities exist that even the mildest cases must be regarded as serious and carefully watched, since we can never know when unfavourable symptoms may develop." For Holt, then, pediatricians' professional duties required them to be fully informed about the bacteriological basis of a diphtheria diagnosis and also to recognize that *Corynebacterium diphtheriae* was capable of manifesting in a range of bodily symptoms.[10]

Because diphtheria was highly contagious, the need to prevent its spread to healthy children remained an urgent imperative. As sanitarians turned their attention away from controlling the foul environmental miasmas they had once held responsible for generating epidemic diseases such as cholera, typhoid, and yellow fever, new techniques for identifying and measuring pathogens pointed to possible bacterial dangers lurking in local water and milk supplies. Improving laboratory techniques enabled public health departments, particularly those in larger cities, to gather and analyze data in the effort to trace sources of bacteriological contamination. Precisely identifying such sources, it was hoped, could lead to the eradication of a number of deadly childhood diseases. The epidemiological approach held out a particular promise for assuaging the ever-present childhood scourge of diarrheal diseases known as cholera infantum, or summer complaint. Pasteurization of milk was being used in Europe and would soon be introduced in the United States as well. But diphtheria was different. Rather than residing in a single source of contamination, the bacterium that caused it likely inhabited the mucous membranes of tens of thousands of people, including many who were not exhibiting obvious symptoms of infection. Without a definitive understanding of its etiology, diphtheria's prevention remained elusive.[11]

Prior to the late nineteenth century, available options for containing the spread of deadly diseases had been limited to severe measures such as enacting strict quarantines, forcibly removing sick people (including children) out of the general population and into the local "pest house," and, in the case of smallpox, mandating vaccination—all of which were regularly met with resistance from alarmed members of the public. Armed with new bacteriological evidence, public health officials gained even more authority over individuals whose very bodies were now coming under scrutiny as vectors transferring disease. In many areas throughout the United States, however, resistance to the intrusiveness of public health departments remained robust. Nor was the regular medical community itself immediately united in accepting the validity of a theory that posited vaguely understood germs as the root cause of illness over evidence that was easily observable in the environment such as foul odors and dampness. Although by the 1890s most regular physicians endorsed a greater role for the laboratory sciences, many remained concerned about public health officials' overreach, pointing out that harsh actions were perceived a punitive by the public and often frightened sick people away from seeking the medical help they desperately needed. Further, if diseases were now to be defined bacteriologically rather than symptomatically, what might be the consequences for the so-called "healthy carriers" whose bodies harbored dangerous bacilli but who were not themselves sick? Some researchers countered that increasingly precise knowledge of how infectious diseases spread could allow for responses that were both less severe and more effective in protecting the public's health. In 1893 William H. Park argued that his portable method, which enabled physicians to get laboratory confirmation within a matter of hours, would actually soften the impact of public health interventions because "no suspicious case that is not diphtheria [will] be regarded and treated as such any longer than the fourteen hours absolutely necessary for making the diagnosis." Trusting his own diagnostic system, Park imagined that community cooperation in safeguarding the public's health might actually be enhanced when official actions were guided by the logic of the laboratory.[12]

Leading pediatricians in the United States, notably both the specialty's pioneer Abraham Jacobi and its influential second-generation educator Luther Emmett Holt, favored strong public health responses in the effort to control the spread of diphtheria. In 1897 Holt, who by this time had held more than half a dozen positions at various medical institutions for children as well as maintaining a private pediatric practice, warned physicians that the bacillus could be transmitted by inhaling the breath of infected children and coming into contact with discharges from their saliva and mucous; even commonplace actions such as touching a sick child's toy, spoon, or drinking cup posed a potential threat. He did not shy away from noting that seemingly healthy adults who came into close contact with children— including medical practitioners—unwittingly contributed to diphtheria's spread, pointedly noting that "the frequency of diphtheria in physicians' families bears witness to the great danger of infection." Holt pointed out that the very tools doctors employed in their ministrations to sick children, including tongue depressors, cotton wool, and the instruments used in tracheotomy and intubation, harbored multiple strains of deadly bacteria. To minimize their own exposure he advised pediatricians to place a pane of window glass between their own faces and those of their young patients. Holt provided a sobering assessment of diphtheria's spread and he advocated forceful actions during local outbreaks such as bans on public funerals for diphtheria victims, closing down schools, and barring children who lived in households where the disease was present from participating in any public activities. He insisted that "not only every undoubted case of diphtheria, but every suspected case must be isolated." Given the logistical difficulty of separating sick children who lived in crowded tenement buildings from their families and neighbors, Holt argued that such children must be removed from their homes entirely and placed in hospital isolation wards where their contact with other people would be severely restricted. "The quarantine in every instance must be complete," he maintained. "No person should be allowed in the room except the attendants and the physician. The meals and everything else required by the patient must be left outside the door." As long as prevention remained the best weapon available for combatting diphtheria's deadly spread, influential pediatricians such as Holt viewed these bleak scenarios as the best hope for saving many children's lives.[13]

In 1897, however, Holt could point to a new option: diphtheria antitoxin, a remedy that had only recently, and quite dramatically, engaged the attention of the regular medical community. Beginning in 1890 researchers in Berlin and Paris had experimented with stimulating immunity to diphtheria in animals by using an antitoxin derived from the blood sera of other animals already immune to the disease. Paul Ehrlich of the Robert Koch Institute discovered a method for producing a more effective diphtheria antitoxin, and in December 1891 a child in Berlin became the first human patient to be treated with the experimental therapy. Three years later Pierre Paul Émile Roux, the highly respected bacteriologist, physician, and co-founder of the Pasteur Institute, reported that using antitoxin had reduced the number of diphtheria deaths in a Paris hospital by half. Roux's announcement, given at an international medical conference in Budapest, bestowed the imprimatur of scientific credibility upon the new approach and support for this promising new direction burgeoned. In London the Wellcome Research Laboratories and the British Institute of Preventive Medicine began producing serum and distributing it widely, including exporting it to clinics and hospitals in the United States. In January 1895 the New York City Health Department began distributing serum manufactured by its own laboratory under the direction of William H. Park. The following year the American Pediatric Society commissioned a study to assess physicians' use of antitoxin in private practice. The results from 5800 reported cases were extremely encouraging, showing that only 12.3%

of children treated with serum therapy had died; when antitoxin was administered within three days of the disease's onset, mortality fell to just 7.3%. Despite ongoing scientific disagreements about the nature of diphtheria itself, after 1896 the regular medical community in the United States widely supported the new remedy. Abraham Jacobi endorsed the use of antitoxin while at the same time warning physicians not to abandon their established knowledge and experience for an exclusively bacteriological approach to understanding and treating the disease.[14]

Luther Emmett Holt's influential volume *The Diseases of Infancy and Childhood*, which arrived just one year after the commission released its report, reflected pediatricians' cautious optimism. The text included graphs indicating strikingly steep declines in the number of reported diphtheria deaths in New York, Chicago, Newark, and Boston following the introduction of antitoxin in those cities. But physicians could also observe the new therapy's benefits first-hand. When administered promptly, Holt explained, antitoxin's benefits became apparent very quickly, with observable improvement taking place within twelve to twenty-four hours of injection. A sufferer's fever and pulse rate subsided, there was a rapid reduction in the redness and swelling of the mucous membranes, discharges dried up, and the stupor and restless movements that were characteristic of the most severe cases mercifully ceased. The pseudomembrane ceased spreading and then became soft and loose enough to be easily expelled. But, even as he described these stunning salutary effects, Holt cautioned that antitoxin was not a panacea. He noted that the available research suggested that the new therapy was most effective in younger rather than older children. Further, it was absolutely critical to administer the serum within forty-eight hours of diphtheria's onset, before bacterial toxins irreparably damaged a patient's kidneys, nervous system, or heart. Finally, even when antitoxin cured diphtheria, Holt cautioned that patients could still die from other causes, including the streptococcus infections often associated with diphtheria cases. Like Jacobi, Holt asserted that antitoxin should be regarded as a complement to, rather than a replacement for, existing therapeutic practices.[15]

As research institutions in England, Germany, and the United States went forward with the production and distribution of serum, public health officials were notably less reserved than were pediatricians in voicing their enthusiasm for the new therapy. In 1895 Hermann M. Biggs of the New York Health Department, which was itself garnering public support for a plan to produce and distribute antitoxin free of charge, claimed that the serum was "apparently devoid of injurious effects, [and] may be administered without any apprehension as to the results." Despite Biggs' confidence, antitoxin's transition from the laboratory to a standard remedy for diphtheria did not take a straightforward path. While early reports of its effectiveness were indeed very positive, gathering accurate data outside of hospitals and clinics was complicated by the fact that the number of diphtheria deaths in the United States naturally fluctuated from year to year. What is more, safe dosages and potency levels for the remedy had yet to be determined. Cases of "serum sickness" (severe and even lethal reactions immediately after antitoxin was administered) and skin eruptions at the site of injection were reported at scientific conferences and in the pages of medical journals. Further, in the drive to produce antitoxin quickly and in large quantities, the specter of improperly manufactured or contaminated serum represented a potential public health crisis of its own; the first of several such disasters, in fact, would occur in St. Louis in 1901. Last, but by no means least important, the dilemma remained unresolved as to whether antitoxin should routinely be administered to the thousands, and perhaps even millions, of "healthy carriers"—individuals who harbored *Cornynebacterium diphtheriae* in their mucous membranes but exhibited no symptoms of the disease. Toward that end, medical researchers in both Europe and the United States explored the possible use of antitoxin to preemptively immunize populations, an effort that continued into the first decades of the twentieth century.[16]

To be truly effective in controlling diphtheria, public health measures such as the mandatory reporting of cases, imposing quarantines where diphtheria was detected, and employing governmental agencies to produce and distribute antitoxin required a significant degree of cooperation from the individuals and communities affected—particularly from the parents of children whose lives might be spared by these efforts. Thus information concerning these rapid and far-reaching changes in scientific medicine needed to extend well beyond the academic and technical debates taking place within the public health and regular medical communities. Because diphtheria was an endemic disease that predictably killed thousands of children each year in the United States, local outbreaks did not necessarily constitute "news" and therefore the popular press had not devoted much space to discussing the disease prior to the late nineteenth century. In the mid-1890s, however, the academic excitement surrounding antitoxin spilled over into coverage of both the new bacteriological understanding of diphtheria and the promising new therapy in mass-market magazines and daily local newspapers. Seeking widespread support for their ambitious initiatives, urban public health officials themselves produced much of the pro-antitoxin material that was then replicated in the popular press.[17]

In March 1895 the New York Health Department, in partnership with the *New York Herald*, launched a subscription drive in support of the manufacture and distribution of antitoxin for use in the city's poor districts where the disease was believed to be most prevalent. That month the nationally circulated *McClure's Magazine* featured pieces by Hermann M. Biggs and William H. Park that translated the latest information about diphtheria to an urban and middle-class readership nationwide. "If a visitor should stop at our laboratory any morning at an earlier hour," Park explained in a generously illustrated article, "he would notice a large number of little tubes containing sterilized blood serum." After thus inviting the reader into the obscure and somewhat shadowy world of the laboratory, Park described the damage done to the human body by diphtheria's bacteriological toxins. The piece finished with a description of the process by which antitoxin was procured using blood serum obtained from immunized horses. While Park's essay was simple yet substantive, city newspapers with less print space to spare often printed brief, rather cryptic, items taken from wire services. In December 1895, for example, the *Chicago Inter-Ocean* devoted a column and a half to discussing in some detail the statistical results of antitoxin studies recently conducted in New York City. The information was of interest to Chicago readers, the editors explained, because Chicago's Department of Public Health was currently using antitoxin produced by New York City's laboratory. The piece concluded by reporting that the eminent bacteriologist William H. Welch of Johns Hopkins University, who had reviewed recent studies from both Europe and the United States and concluded "beyond a reasonable doubt that anti-diphtheric serum is a specific curative agent for diphtheria, surpassing in its efficacy all other known methods of treatment of the disease." In the ensuing weeks, newspapers such as the *Pittsburgh Dispatch* and the *Emporia* (Kansas) *Daily Gazette* picked up and reprinted Welch's quote, but eliminated the contextual information that would help readers make sense of his statement. In addition to reportage and wire services, explications of bacteriology and antitoxin sometimes came from local physicians in the form of letters to the editor. Most enigmatic, and doubtlessly confusing for the general reading public, were advertisements placed by local pharmacies that announced the availability of diphtheria antitoxin directly alongside promotions for patent medicines promising to cure all manner of ailments from malaria to tuberculosis.[18]

A consistent feature of mainstream press coverage was its unquestioning acceptance of regular medicine's scientific authority. In many states, regular physicians were engaged in fierce political battles with sectarian practitioners over new statutory requirements for medical education and licensing. Sociologist Owen Whooley has challenged the notion that the medical revolution engendered by the laboratory sciences naturally and inevitably favored "allopathic" physicians over their homeopathic competitors. Rather, he argues, regulars actively forged ties to European bacteriologists through training and scholarly exchanges that allowed them to lay claim to each new advancement. Over the following decades, as bacteriology came to dominate western medicine, homeopaths' continued skepticism of the germ theory would prove to be professionally fatal. In the 1890s this contest played out in the popular press as the two schools debated the causes of diphtheria as well as the safety and efficacy of antitoxin. In Chicago, where the American Medical Association was headquartered, the *Daily Tribune* printed rebuttal letters from homeopathic physicians that challenged the paper's optimistic reporting on the promise of the new bacteriological theories. A letter from a reader named Dr. R. N. Hooker, for example, declared that "the germ theory is fallacious" because "in a large portion of cases of indisputable diphtheria the [Klebs-Loeffler] bacillus is absent." The writer then provided data garnered from his own survey purporting to demonstrate that "homeopathy shows a record in the treatment of this disease which is better than the anti-toxin three to one." Homeopaths also vehemently opposed the Chicago Board of Health's aggressive promotion of antitoxin as an intrusion into their own professional prerogatives. In October 1895 the Board initiated a new policy to tackle diphtheria in the city. At the request of attending physicians, health officials would bring antitoxin directly to suspected diphtheria cases. Physicians then had the choice of administering the injections themselves or, alternatively, requesting it be done by the health officials. In addition to the injections, a specimen would be taken and returned to the city's pathology laboratory for confirmation. Both the antitoxin and the laboratory work were offered free of charge, but physicians were obligated to file a report of each case with the Board of Health (presumably for accounting, and perhaps epidemiological, purposes). The plan's final provision made antitoxin available at stations located throughout the city for doctors to purchase at low cost. Homeopathic practitioners, who were eligible for medical licenses under existing Illinois law, bristled at this unprecedented professional partnership with the Chicago Board of Health. "I am opposed to its coming between families and their physicians," declared C. E. Fisher of the Illinois Homeopathic Medical Society, "and trying to destroy the practice of men who are a hundred times better and more skillful physicians than any in the [public health] department." Like most of his colleagues, Fisher dismissed diphtheria antitoxin as nothing more than a passing "fad."[19]

Meanwhile, as theoretical disagreements embroiled researchers and practitioners of scientific and sectarian medicine, parents faced bewildering and perhaps even agonizing decisions about how to help their sick children. In the 1890s, bacteriology represented a very recent reimagining of a frightening disease, and its implications for any particular child's case remained uncertain. Children suffering from an ailment that appeared to be diphtheria sometimes recovered, but sometimes they did not. As the Jacobis unfortunately learned, the illness could take sudden and unexpected turns for the worse, even under the watchful eyes of highly educated and fully informed parents. O'Dwyer's new intubation method, while less dangerous than tracheotomy, was nevertheless stressful for the child and quite disturbing for parents to witness. And, if the much-discussed new serum therapy offered promise, it also came with real risks and uncertainties of its own. Amid all this confusion, then, it is not hard to imagine that a complete rejection of scientific medicine, framed as a higher and eternal truth not subject to the imperfect knowledge of mere mortal beings, might offer succor and hope to distraught parents. "One disease is just as much a delusion as another," Mary Baker Eddy wrote in 1893—the same year that visitors to the World's Columbian Exposition in Chicago viewed a bacteriological exhibit featuring *Cornynebacterium diphtheriae* growing in a test tube. "It is a pity that the medical faculty and clergy have not found this out." The founder of Christian Science provided her followers with an alternative explanation for the cause of their children's distressing physical symptoms. "I have discovered disease in the human mind, and recognized the fear of it," she wrote, "many weeks before the so-called disease made an appearance in the human body." Because the *thought* of illness preceded its corporeal manifestations, she continued, "faith in the rules of health or of drugs begets and fosters disease." Regardless of the current excitement over bacteriology and the new remedies being promoted by medical science and the popular press, Eddy insisted to her followers that "we should put no faith in material means."[20]

Importantly for Eddy, regular medicine was not merely useless in curing disease. Those who practiced it, she warned, actually caused harm through the fear they spread when they attached names to what were only illusory bodily symptoms and, even further, when they reported those names to local authorities. Public health officials then escalated the danger by placing a household under quarantine and attaching a placard carrying the named disease on a door or window, perpetuating fear in anyone who happened to view it. "We weep because others weep, we yawn because they yawn, and we have smallpox because others have it," Eddy wrote, in her church's foundation text, *Science and Health with Key to the Scriptures*. "Mortal mind, not matter, carries the infection." In a published essay entitled "Contagion," Eddy asserted that "People believe in contagious diseases, and that anyone is liable to have them under certain predisposing or exciting causes. This mental state prepares one to have any disease whenever there appear the circumstances which he believes to produce it." Thus the same public health measures that the regular medical community regarded as essential for controlling outbreaks of diphtheria and other childhood scourges —disseminating information on the latest medical science, reporting infectious disease to local health officials, and placing infected individuals under quarantine—represented the worst sort of folly to Christian Scientists. Perhaps not surprisingly then, the church's healers soon found themselves running afoul of the law by refusing to report cases of infectious disease in violation of public health ordinances. They also gained notoriety for their practice of entering "sin and fear" as causes of death on official certificates, prompting several states to ban Christian Science healers from signing the documents in the role of attending medical practitioner.[21]

Tensions between Christian Scientists and public health authorities are well illustrated in an 1898 report published in the *Christian Science Journal*, the official church publication that regularly featured accounts of successful healings through metaphysical means. In the account from Washington, DC, a young boy had been suffering from diphtheria. His desperate parents contacted a Christian Science healer, who arrived to find the child "in great suffering, and the family in sore distress of mind and fear." The healer then applied the procedure of mentally arguing away the parents' belief that their little boy was ill, replacing such thoughts with the understanding that their child was in perfect health. Soon the pseudomembrane spontaneously ejected from the child's throat, allowing him to breathe freely and rest quietly. Trouble arose, however, when a public health official arrived at the home and placed a placard marked "diphtheria" outside the house. The official then menaced the Christian Science healer, warning her that "if the worse comes, as is likely, it will probably be very unpleasant for you." Such a rebuke frightened the healer and she left the scene. Unfortunately, with the diphtheria label now attached to the household and the healer no longer ministering to the child's parents, "malicious error" seeped in and the child died within just a few hours. Despite this sad conclusion, however, the account's author promoted the case as a successful demonstration of Christian Science healing. She noted that the child had "passed without any of the suffering or distress usual in such cases under physicians"—a likely reference to the exigencies of intubation and perhaps the injection of antitoxin. The lesson was not that the boy died, but rather that he had been spared unnecessary torment at the hands of medical doctors. The report did not indicate whether the health official made good on his threat to hold the healer liable in the child's death. Elsewhere, however, Christian Science practitioners did endure harsh treatment by public health authorities. In at least one reported case a female healer apparently was entrapped by a man pretending to be sick. When outbreaks of diphtheria spiked, as they commonly did in the late nineteenth century, Christian Scientists blamed the regular medicine community for spreading fear while health officials fingered Eddy and her followers for willfully and recklessly endangering both the public's health and children's lives.[22]

Newspapers reported frequently, and usually sensationally, on the deaths of children under the care of Christian Science healers. "Killed by Faith and Neglect," ran a typically lurid headline. In 1898, for example, six-year-old Lillian Lewis died of diphtheria in her Chicago home. (While it was headquartered in Boston, Christian Science was gaining a significant following in the Midwest, particularly in Chicago.) The *Chicago Daily Tribune* quoted the Cook County coroner's blunt assertion calling the little girl's death "one of the worst cases of neglect that ever came under my observation." His postmortem examination had determined, the paper graphically noted, that Lillian had slowly choked to death while the pseudomembrane filled her throat. Further, he found that "the healthy condition of the other organs is good evidence that the child might have been saved by a medical operation" (presumably a reference to tracheotomy or intubation). Tensions in Chicago escalated as the American Medical Association weighed into the public debate with a series of strong denouncements of Mary Baker Eddy individually, and of her followers collectively, in the pages of its official organ, the *Journal of the American Medical Association*. "Steps should be taken to restrain the rabid utterances and the irrational practices of such ignorant and irresponsible persons," the journal railed in a characteristic diatribe. Such vitriol was not entirely unusual for the *Journal of the American Medical Association* at the turn of the twentieth century. At this time the American Medical Association was lobbying aggressively in Illinois to have that state's legislature expressly outlaw, not only Christian Science healing, but also the faith-healing practices of the Christian Catholic Apostolic Church, a militantly anti-medical church founded by John Alexander Dowie that was also headquartered in Chicago and had also begun to attract a national following.[23]

Like the public controversy engendered by the Abby Corner case a decade earlier, Christian Scientists' continued run-ins with public health authorities threw into sharp relief the dilemma of reconciling a metaphysical health care paradigm predicated on a complete rejection of medical science with the growing social and political authority of regular medicine. And again, Eddy ultimately resolved the impasse by modifying one of her church's core tenets. In 1902, in what scholar Shawn Francis Peters has described as a "startling turnabout" on her position regarding the dangers of spreading illness by cooperating with public health authorities, Eddy informed her followers that "until public thought becomes better acquainted with Christian Science," the church's practitioners would be required to report cases of contagious disease to local officials when the law required them to do so. Even further, the faithful must vaccinate their children against smallpox in compliance with state or local mandates. "I have always believed that Christian Scientists should be law abiding," she asserted. By the time of her death in 1910, Eddy would extend her compromise with regular medicine several more times, allowing her followers to seek regular medical assistance in the repair of broken bones, the performance of dental work, the correction of vision with eyeglasses, and the administration of morphine for the relief of pain. But, while the new directive distanced the organizational church from potential legal liability, it left unresolved the underlying problem for the faithful who sincerely believed that their own fearful thoughts could transmit bodily sickness to their children. The state might mandate the reporting of contagious disease cases, but Christian Scientist parents still risked their children's lives if they acknowledged bodily symptoms and sought the aid of medical practitioners other than the healers trained and certified by their church.[24]

Even as the prestige of bacteriology grew, the inability to cure most infectious diseases once they had been contracted meant that prevention remained the most powerful weapon in saving children's lives. The pathology laboratory had revealed that the cause of many dangerous ailments was bacteria carried in water and milk supplies and transferred by close human contact. In the early twentieth century pediatricians allied with child welfare advocates in a number of ambitious initiatives to prevent the spread of bacterial diseases, especially the diarrheal diseases that continued to threaten the health of thousands of children each year. In 1909 the alliance formally organized as the American Association for the Study and Prevention of Infant Mortality based in New Haven, Connecticut. Several major cities created special divisions within their public health departments dedicated to initiatives aimed at preventing the spread of the bacterial diseases of childhood. The first was New York City's Bureau of Child Hygiene led by physician S. Josephine Baker, whose aggressive efforts included dispatching public health nurses to visit the homes of the poor armed with information and advice on practices such as bathing babies daily and frequent handwashing by adults.[25]

If parental education and persuasion represented one approach to saving children's lives at the turn of the twentieth century, the use of the law represented another. An expansion of the concept of child neglect led a number of states to legally require parents to seek the services of regular medical practitioners for conditions now regarded as treatable. In 1905, the United States Supreme Court rejected the Reverend Henning Jacobson's argument that a Massachusetts statute violated his liberty interest in deciding, for his child as well as for himself, whether to undergo vaccination during a smallpox outbreak in Boston and Cambridge. Writing for the majority, Justice John Marshall Harlan accepted as axiomatic that vaccination was an effective means of preventing the spread of smallpox. Five years after the *Jacobson* ruling, the influential Judge Harvey Baker of the Boston juvenile court asserted that his state's criminal medical neglect statutes encompassed parents' failure to prevent ophthalmia neonatorum and bowed shinbones in their children—ailments that by 1910 had become medically treatable. Even further, in a number of states parents who refused to seek regular medical services for their dying children on the basis of their religious beliefs now faced the threat of criminal prosecution.[26]

## NOTES

1. "Bottled Up Death," *Chicago Daily Tribune* (May 17, 1893): 9; Samuel H. Preston and Michael R. Haines, *Fatal Years: Child Mortality in*

*Late Nineteenth-Century America* (Princeton: Princeton University Press, 1991), 5.

2. Arthur E. Hertzler, *The Horse and Buggy Doctor* (New York: Harper and Brothers, 1939), 3; A. Jacobi, *A Treatise on Diphtheria* (New York: William Wood and Company, 1880), 68–107.

3. Evelynn Maxine Hammonds, *Childhood's Deadly Scourge: The Campaign to Control Diphtheria in New York City, 1880–1930* (Baltimore: Johns Hopkins University Press, 1999), 30–36.

4. Jacobi, *Treatise on Diphtheria*, 151–234; Harry F. Dowling, *Fighting Infection: Conquests of the Twentieth Century* (Cambridge, MA: Harvard University Press, 1977), 19.

5. Joseph O'Dwyer, *Intubation in Croup and Other Acute and Chronic Forms of Stenosis of the Larynx* (New York: William Wood and Company, 1889), 272–278; Anne Hardy, "Tracheotomy Versus Intubation: Surgical Intervention in Diphtheria in Europe and the United States, 1825–1930," *Bulletin of the History of Medicine*, Volume 66 (1992): 536–559.

6. Hammonds, *Childhood's Deadly Scourge*, 28–36; Rhonda Truax, *The Doctors Jacobi* (Boston: Little, Brown, 1952), 197–199.

7. Hammonds, *Childhood's Deadly Scourge*, 30; A. Jacobi, "Diphtheria Spread by Adults," *New York Medical Journal*, Volume XL (September 27, 1884): 344–347.

8. John Duffy, *From Humors to Medical Science: A History of American Medicine*. Second edition (Urbana: University of Illinois Press, 1993), 167–187; George Rosen, *A History of Public Health*. Revised expanded edition (Baltimore: Johns Hopkins University Press, 2015), 184–199; Owen Whooley, *Knowledge in the Time of Cholera* (Chicago: University of Chicago Press, 2013), 183–220.

9. Hammonds, *Childhood's Deadly Scourge*, 58–64, 75–87; William Hallock Park, "Diphtheria and Other Pseudomembranous Inflammations—A Clinical and Bacteriological Study," *New York Medical Record*, Volume 43, Number 6 (Winter 1893): 161–168; Rosen, *A History of Public Health*, 189–190.

10. Luther Emmett Holt, *The Diseases of Infancy and Childhood* (New York: D. Appleton and Company, 1897), 950–980.

11. Park, "Diphtheria and Other Pseudomembranous Inflammations," 168.

12. On popular resistance to public health authority at the turn of the twentieth century, see Judith Walzer Leavitt, *Typhoid Mary: Captive to the Public's Health* (Boston: Beacon Press, 1996); Robert D. Johnston, *The Radical Middle Class: Populist Democracy and the Question of Capitalism in Progressive Era Portland, Oregon* (Princeton, NJ: Princeton University Press, 2003); Nadav Davidovitch, "Negotiating Dissent: Homeopathy and Anti-Vaccinationism at the Turn of the Twentieth Century."

In Robert D. Johnston, editor, *The Politics of Healing: Histories of Alternative Medicine in Twentieth-Century North America* (New York and London: Routledge, 2004), 11–28; Michael Willrich, *Pox: An American History* (New York: Penguin Press, 2011); Karen L. Walloch, *The Antivaccine Heresy: Jacobson v. Massachusetts and the Troubled History of Compulsory Vaccination in the United States* (Rochester, NY: University of Rochester Press, 2015).

13. Holt, *The Diseases of Infancy and Childhood*, 954, 982; Sydney A. Halpern, *American Pediatrics* (Berkeley: University of California Press, 1988), 55–62.

14. Rosen, *A History of Public Health*, 189–194; Dowling, *Fighting Infection*, 36–43; H. J. Parish, *A History of Immunization* (Edinburgh: E. and S. Livingstone, 1965), 119–125; Hammonds, *Childhood's Deadly Scourge*, 132–137.

15. Holt, *The Diseases of Infancy and Childhood*, 988–1001.

16. Hermann M. Biggs, "The New Treatment of Diphtheria," *McClure's Magazine*, Volume IV, Number 4 (March 1895): 360–364; Paul Weindling, "From Research to Clinical Practice: Serum Therapy for Diphtheria in the 1890s." In John V. Pickstone, editor, *Medical Innovations in Historical Perspective* (New York: St. Martin's Press, 1992), 72–83.

17. Terra Ziporyn, *Disease in the Popular Press: The Case of Diphtheria, Typhoid Fever, and Syphilis, 1870–1920* (New York: Greenwood Press, 1988), 39–46.

18. William H. Park, "Diphtheria Antitoxine—Its Production," *McClure's Magazine*, Volume IV, Number 4 (March 1895): 365–369; "Use of Antitoxin," *Chicago Inter-Ocean* (December 16, 1895): 11.

19. Whooley, *Knowledge in the Time of Cholera*, 154; "Plan to Lower City's Death Rate," *Chicago Daily Tribune* (October 6, 1895): 9; "Dr. R. N. Tooker Gives Reasons," *Chicago Daily Tribune* (January 13, 1896): 7; "Will Go to the Public," *Chicago Daily Tribune* (January 11, 1896): 7.

20. Mary Baker Eddy, *Science and Health with Key to the Scriptures*, Seventy-seventh edition, revised (Boston: E. J. Foster Eddy, 1893), 294, 61–62.

21. Eddy, *Science and Health* (1893), 47; Mary Baker Eddy, "Contagion." In *Miscellaneous Writings 1883–1896* (Boston: Allison V. Stewart, 1916), 228–229; Rennie B. Schoepflin, *Christian Science on Trial: Religious Healing in America* (Baltimore: Johns Hopkins University Press, 2003), 101–106; "Magnetic Healers," *Journal of the American Medical Association*, Volume 33 (October 1899): 92.

22. "That Case in Washington, D.C.," *Christian Science Journal*, Volume 16 (June 1898): 187–188.

23. "Killed by Faith and Neglect," *Chicago Daily Tribune* (April 22, 1888): 3; "Killed by Christian Science," *The Quincy Daily Journal* (October 12, 1892): 1; "Christian Science Fails to Save Life of Lillian Lewis," *Chicago*

*Daily Tribune* (October 23, 1899): 12; "Say Repeal If Akin Is Right," *Chicago Daily Tribune* (September 10, 1899): 8; "The Immorality of Christian Science," *Journal of the American Medical Association*, Volume 33 (November 18, 1899): 1299.

24. Shawn Francis Peters, *When Prayer Fails: Faith Healing, Children, and the Law* (New York: Oxford University Press, 2008), 95; Schoepflin, *Christian Science on Trial*, 80; Gottschalk, *Rolling Away the Stone*, 350–351.

25. Richard A. Meckel, *Save the Babies: American Public Health Reform and the Prevention of Infant Mortality, 1850–1929* (Baltimore: Johns Hopkins University Press, 1990), 62–91; S. Josephine Baker, *Fighting for Life* (1939; Reprinted by the New York Review of Books, 2013), 82–87.

26. *Jacobsen v. Massachusetts* 197 U.S. 11 (1905); Linda Gordon, *Heroes of Their Own Lives: The Politics and History of Family Violence* (Penguin Books, 1988), 127–129.

# CHAPTER 6

# Children on the Battle Line Between Religion and Medicine

Has the law a right to come in and interfere with your children, and say you have no right to forbid those children receiving medicine? Can doctors claim the right by law to open your child's mouth and thrust this or that medicine down its throat, whether you like it or not?

In 1900 John Alexander Dowie exhorted parents to join with him in a religious crusade against practitioners of scientific medicine. "This is becoming a fight between the Devil and Drugs on one side and God and Divine Healing on the Other," he thundered in a self-published circular, *Zion's Holy War Against the Hosts of Hell in Chicago.* "Every time I capture a doctor's deadly instruments, I am happy." Sickness and injury came from the devil, he preached, and sinful behavior provided the opening through which evil entered to torment the human body. Thus only God had the power to heal. But Dowie also claimed he could channel divine healing power through the medium of his own hands. In 1877, during an epidemic raging in Newtown, Australia, the Scottish-born minister discovered the power to heal was "in my hands, and in my hands I hold it still, and I will never lay it down." Separating from the Congregational Church, he founded an independent ministry upon his newly discovered gift. In 1890, as president of the International Divine Healing Association, Dowie arrived in Chicago and began holding religious services that featured miraculous

© The Author(s) 2019
L. Curry, *Religion, Law, and the Medical Neglect of Children in the United States, 1870–2000,*
Palgrave Studies in the History of Childhood,
https://doi.org/10.1007/978-3-030-24689-1_6

cures. He soon caught the attention of the local press, which mocked his odd speech and wild gestures and disparaged his unsophisticated followers. Dowie resembled "a man fighting a windmill," the *Chicago Daily Tribune* chortled, noting that each service began with the passing of the collection plate; the naïfs seeking cures belonged to the "class of persons that jumps backward from a moving car." Despite his rough treatment by the press, Dowie persevered in Chicago and on May 7, 1893 he opened Zion Tabernacle, a small wooden structure located just outside of the 62nd Street entrance gate to the World's Columbian Exposition, directly across from Buffalo Bill's Wild West Show. He pronounced his own mission a resounding success, claiming that some twenty thousand people had found their way to the little wooden church to be cured of their ailments. Declaring that he still had work to do in Chicago, the divine healer stayed on in that city after the fair closed in the fall.[1]

The following year Dowie resumed publication of *Leaves of Healing*, a periodical he had started in San Francisco before he relocated to the Midwest, in order to spread the word of his religious mission far beyond the Chicago environs. In each issue much space was devoted to descriptions of the healing services held at the original Zion Tabernacle, and soon at the two additional churches Dowie established on the west and north sides of the city. Distressed parents of sick and injured children learned of special rites held for their little ones. Dowie described hundreds of children crowding into the little church, "piling up and piling up on mothers' knees, and often two in a chair." After delivering a sermon appropriately pitched for a child's understanding, Dowie elicited personal testimonials from "many whose little legs have been lengthened, deaf and dumb who can now speak and hear, some who have never walked from birth who can now walk and leap and run" because they had received the gift of his blessing. If such words did not prove convincing enough to parents of sick children, photographs powerfully enhanced the divine healer's message. In August 1894, Willie Esser attested to the instantaneous healing of his leg by Dowie, a miracle the ten-year-old experienced only after enduring years of unsuccessful treatment by "many doctors in the city." A formal studio portrait depicted a demure boy smartly dressed in a suit and straw hat, his hands holding up the crutch and iron leg brace upon which he had once depended to walk. Elsewhere in the issue readers could view an arresting image showing a collection of discarded prostheses mounted on one wall of Zion Tabernacle; the caption below it read, "Captured From the Enemy." Parents learned that, if they held strong in the faith, their children would have no need for drugs or devices. "If you are sick let the spirit of God flow through your whole body," Dowie promised. "Open wide the gates. If you do there will be no further use for crutches or spectacles, and no more pains and aches."[2]

But Dowie did not limit his divine healing mission to restoring children's damaged limbs. *Leaves of Healing* also regularly described his gift for ridding children of various diseases, including those that the new science of bacteriology hoped to eradicate. An issue published in April 1897 carried the story of Mabel Bush, an eight-year-old girl whom Dowie had cured of diphtheria. Sadly, however, the little girl was subsequently "killed by the injection of Anti-Toxine [sic] by Doctors representing the Board of Health" who refused to accept the word of the little girl's parents that the disease had been driven from their child's body by the divine healer's gift. The new serum therapy had arrived in Chicago in 1895 via a city ordinance that also provided the substantial sum of $10,000 to purchase antitoxin from the New York City Department of Public Health, allowing physicians to procure it at low cost for use in their private practices. For Dowie, the widespread use of antitoxin, subsidized by public funds, was a monstrous folly. He warned parents that Chicago's antitoxin plan was only the beginning of a tyrannical plot to erode their freedom to choose religious over secular healing. The Illinois state legislature, he charged, intended to "hand their children over as slaves to the professional poisoners." In a defiant gesture toward the Chicago health authorities, Dowie mounted a vial of diphtheria antitoxin on the Zion Tabernacle wall, placing it among the motley collection of crutches, braces, plaster casts, and modified shoes regularly used by physicians to torment the bodies of children.[3]

Today John Alexander Dowie is best remembered among historians of religion for his radical ministry that broke with the broader divine healing movement of the nineteenth century and presaged the emergence of Pentecostalism in the early twentieth.[4] Historian Timothy E. W. Gloege has argued that the brief but incendiary conflict between Dowie and the medical community of Illinois reflected wider struggles for moral authority among competing members of an emerging professional class in the United States, a pattern noted by other scholars. Ronald L. Numbers, for example, examined the complex professional relationship between Seventh-Day Adventism's founder Ellen G. White and the physician and health reformer John Harvey Kellogg. In a partnership that was both long and productive, White frequently revised her pronouncements on health and medicine, which her followers regarded as prophecy, so that they aligned with the latest scientific views coming from Kellogg's laboratories. Nevertheless tensions between White and Kellogg persisted, ending with the latter's total "disfellowship" from the church. In Chicago, the bodies of sick and injured children occupied a significant place in the struggle as Dowie rallied parents to join him in an apocalyptic crusade to beat back the imposition of regular medicine aided by an authoritarian state. The fact that his following, like that of Mary Baker Eddy, grew quickly at the turn of the twentieth century speaks to significant and lingering distrust of regular medicine even as American society at large underwent rapid transformation by science. Historian Robert C. Fuller has noted that, for many Christian denominations, acts of healing "provide an experiential template for proclaiming the presence of Christ in one's life."[5] In some cases, a radical reliance on faith healing alone served as an outward sign of unwavering religious devotion. Risking their own and their family's health was the "key to it all" for followers of Frank Weston Sandford, a religious healer and contemporary of Dowie who established a community of the faithful in Durham, Maine. According to Sandford's biographer Shirley Nelson, the community chose "faith over reason as the method of living their lives and they were proving that they meant it... More was at stake than the healing of a child's limb." Thus for parents who sincerely believed in Dowie's gift rejecting science-based medical help for their sick and injured children became a potent sign of deep and unquestioning commitment to their religious faith. The resultant controversies thrust parents' private decisions into the public arena, sometimes accompanied by a violent backlash. Dowie was attacked in Hammond, Indiana, for example, by an angry crowd who blamed him when a four-year-old child died of diphtheria under the care of a church elder. For his part, Dowie cited incidents of civil unrest as incontrovertible proof that his enemies—among whom he came to count doctors (and the overexcited medical students who led several violent protests against him), the press, and mainline Protestant leaders—colluded to persecute him. He responded by ratcheting up his inflammatory crusading rhetoric in the press and pulpit. "It does not matter whether I am killed or not," he told the congregation at Zion Tabernacle in November 1899. "The blood of the martyrs is the seed of the church." The more urgent threat, he insisted, were unjust laws that made "every citizen of the State of Illinois a victim of those doctors, who have the power to take our lives."[6]

Although the divine healer's histrionic rhetoric seethed with class resentment, his crusade resists easy characterization solely as a populist revolt against professional elites and medical monopolies. While the regular medical community responded aggressively to Dowie's incursions into the healing arena, it was often ordinary citizens who alerted physicians when his followers refused to seek mainstream medical treatment for the sick and injured, particularly when the sufferers were children. In August 1899, for example, the case of eleven-year-old Susie Vedder was brought to authorities' attention by a concerned neighbor who contacted the coroner's office when the child died under the ministrations of an elder in Dowie's new church. In July 1903 a law student sought to have his ailing seventeen-year-old brother removed from the care of their mother, who was a follower of Dowie. In 1906 Rolvix Harlan, a divinity student at the University of Chicago, warned that Dowie used his anti-physician doctrine as a means of control, forcing his followers to rely on his healing hands alone. Harlan was especially critical of Dowie's teaching that failed cures reflected insufficient faith on the part of the sufferer. Growing ever more belligerent in the press and pulpit, the divine healer condemned the local medical establishment, as well as city and county officials who sought to regulate and control his activities. In 1896, he fortified his religious credentials by dissolving the International Divine Healing Association and replacing it with the Christian Catholic Church, naming himself as the new religion's General Overseer. As word of his mission spread beyond the American Midwest offshoots of the church soon emerged in New York and Canada. Dowie's run-ins with secular medical authorities in Chicago continued, however, and in 1901 the divine healer upped the religious ante yet again, declaring himself to be the third incarnation of the prophet Elijah. Dowie's accelerating self-aggrandizement demonstrates that his interest was never to join forces with other sectarian and religious-based practitioners in an effort to democratize the practice of medicine. The divine healer, in fact, had only contempt for his contemporaries in other healing faiths, especially practitioners of Christian Science which he repeatedly denounced as "quackery" and "mere mesmerism" in his sermons and writings.[7]

Interestingly, Dowie's crusading rhetoric expressly drew upon the growing cultural authority of scientific medicine even as he condemned it. As a divinity student at the University of Edinburgh Dowie had served as a hospital chaplain, and he later claimed to have witnessed unspeakable acts of brutality committed by the medical faculty there. In fact, Dowie frequently returned to the theme of medical barbarism in his sermons and writings, relating graphic horror stories of victims who had been failed by the ineffective, or completely botched, ministrations of doctors. In one startling account Dowie claimed to have rescued a young woman who was

"carried away by the wicked doctors at Cook County Hospital" in a das-
tardly plan to "dissect her in the Masonic Temple." He told an audience
at the Chicago Auditorium that he was aware of hundreds of doctors who
had "defiled" and impregnated women and then "killed both mother and
child" via illegal abortions. Given his view that medical science represented
an unalloyed evil, then, it is particularly striking that he consistently referred
to himself, and insisted that others refer to him, by the title "doctor" as
a signifier of his elevated cultural status, despite having no formal medical education. He responded indignantly to implications that he lacked
the appropriate training—and sufficient social standing—to diagnose and
cure sickness. "Now, I think that even my bitterest enemies will see that
if I wanted to get a license I have the intellectual capacity and culture
enough to get a license with very little difficulty," Dowie told readers of
*Leaves of Healing*. "I certainly feel the intellectual equal of some of these
doctors in Chicago." Successful healings now numbered in the thousands,
Dowie asserted, providing ample *prima facie* evidence of his divine gift.
His second-in-command, John Speicher, regularly used his own professional standing as a state-licensed physician to authenticate the stories of
miraculous cures that filled the pages of *Leaves of Healing*. Faith and prayer
might be the only true means of curing the sick, but medical science provided the proof that Dowie's acts of divine healing were real.[8]

Dowie brought his mission to Chicago at the turn of the twentieth century—just as that city was emerging as a national leader in modern medical education and practice. Historians note that Illinois physicians were
among the nation's most aggressive in challenging the legitimacy of alternative medical sects in their state, launching sustained campaigns against
rival practitioners of homeopathy, naturopathy, and osteopathy. Led by the
Chicago-based American Medical Association, new and stricter standards
for licensing medical practitioners and accrediting medical schools enabled
regular practitioners to enhance their own professional status and eliminate many of their sectarian competitors, including various metaphysical
or "magnetic" healers.[9] The Chicago city health commissioner, Arthur R.
Reynolds, vigorously applied existing health ordinances to Dowie's operations and, when those failed to stick, lobbied for more stringent ones.
Reynolds had been brought into the office to oversee the massive and
complex public health arrangements for the World's Columbian Exposition. Although he was still relatively new to his job, he took an aggressive stance in asserting regular physicians' professional prerogatives in
supervising the city's health. In the year 1895 alone no less than forty-

six warrants charged a range of violations stemming from Dowie's divine healing activities including creating a public nuisance, operating unlicensed hospitals, and criminally defrauding patients.[10]

In 1894 Dowie opened the first of several "healing homes" in Hyde Park, the site of the new and prestigious University of Chicago. Writing in the third person, Dowie assured readers of *Leaves of Healing* that the president of the International Divine Healing Association made his own residence in the healing home, where "all its inmates are treated as his private guests." Readers also learned that "the furnishings of the Home are almost entirely new and have cost in all nearly $8000 which the Lord has graciously provided to the uttermost farthing." An accompanying photograph depicted a substantial three-story brick structure with staff and guests neatly lined up across a tidy front lawn. Amid these genteel surroundings, "Dr. Dowie usually meets the guests several times each week for the special healing services." Neighbors, however, reacted with dismay when large numbers of apparently sick and injured people began crowding into their quiet residential street and several concerned residents reported the healing home to the city health commissioner. One man contacted Reynolds because he believed Dowie had defrauded his friend, a railroad engineer named Frank E. King, who had paid the sum of one hundred and thirty dollars for a stay in the healing home only to be turned out without being cured of tuberculosis. (A staff member explained that King was ordered to leave because his incessant coughing disturbed the other guests.) When Dowie consequently stood trial for medical fraud his counsel insisted the statute applied only to purveyors of patent medicines and quack cures, citing as precedent an 1889 case, *State v. Blue Mountain Joe*. The divine healer, by contrast, had only offered a "blessing" to paying guests, not actual medical treatment. But the court found Dowie guilty and ordered him to pay a fine of one hundred dollars. Although he was no stranger to running afoul of the law (he had spent thirty days in a Melbourne city jail for violating an ordinance against street preaching) the divine healer responded with characteristic fury, denouncing the "monstrously unjust" ruling and warning his followers that "it has been made illegal to pray" in the city of Chicago. A Cook County Superior Court judge later threw out the medical fraud penalty but allowed to stand numerous other citations Dowie had sustained in operating the healing homes. The judge sympathetically recommended that he not renew leases on properties in residential areas. Seeing a way to escape his continual legal woes, Dowie consolidated the four establishments into a single facility, the Zion Home, located on Michigan Avenue in the city's South Loop business district. "Zion" became the new church's center as well as the residence of Dowie, his new associate John Speicher, and both men's families. Run-ins with the city health commissioner continued, however. In October 1896, for example, officials tangled with Zion Home attendants who refused to admit them to take a throat culture from a five-year-old child who had fallen ill. The girl's mother had brought the girl with her when she came to the healing home seeking divine healing for pulmonary tuberculosis.[11]

If Dowie's activities caught the attention of the Chicago health commissioner, they came under even more intense scrutiny from the Cook County Coroner's Office. The prominent Danish surgeon Christian Fenger served in the coroner's office as well as on the faculties of several Chicago area medical schools, where he trained a generation of medical examiners. Fenger pioneered postmortem examinations that incorporated the new techniques of laboratory analysis, helping to make pathology a well-developed specialty in Chicago's medical environs. At the turn of the twentieth century Chicago, like many major American cities, was moving toward replacing the traditional coroner's jury with a modern medical examiner's office. Supporters of the plan argued that politically elected coroners overseeing juries made up of community members were subject to bias and corruption and should be replaced with a system solidly based in forensic science.[12] Physicians in the Cook County Coroner's Office asserted their professional prerogatives when, just three months after the Hyde Park healing home's opening, the death of a guest named Julius F. Kellogg came to their attention. Kellogg was a mathematics professor at Northwestern University in the northern suburb of Evanston and also a relative of the physician and health reformer John Harvey Kellogg. Dowie neglected to report the respected academic's death to the coroner's office, arranging instead to have the body taken to Evanston, where it was embalmed despite the absence of a formal certificate listing a cause of death. Although an investigation eventually determined Kellogg had died of natural causes, Dowie's questionable handling of a death in the healing home aroused physicians' misgivings.[13]

Then, in February 1895, a seven-year-old girl named May Van Houten died from diphtheria while under the care of Dowie's new associate, John Speicher. Dismayed neighbors contacted the coroner's office and reported that, although they had observed the child struggling to breathe for four days, her parents had refused to seek medical aid. Unlike Dowie, Speicher did have a license to practice medicine; Illinois law allowed him to obtain certification using a homeopathy degree from Iowa without sitting for qualifying examinations. The Van Houtens initially refused entrance to a physician from the coroner's office, arguing that a death certificate had already been signed by Speicher. Although they soon relented and allowed the physician to examine their child's body, the coroner's office was now made aware that Speicher had been signing death certificates as the attending physician in cases involving Dowie's followers. The office announced it would not accept Speicher's signature as valid and insisted that henceforth all deaths occurring under the auspices of divine healing must be examined by its own physicians. While Christian Fenger's protégés may have doubted the homeopath Speicher's qualifications to medically determine causes of death, they certainly did not trust Dowie's close associate to bring the demise of his followers to the attention of the authorities. One physician told the press he suspected that Dowie had brought Speicher into his operations expressly to cover up divine healing's failures after the death of Julius Kellogg. The press, however, kept a very keen eye on Dowie's activities, reporting on several deaths of children whose parents were church members. In December 1896 a three-year-old girl died under the care of divine healers; her father insisted he had been previously cured of tuberculosis at Dowie's hands. Months later a woman told the press that, although she had taught her grandson that "the only cure was divine healing" the eleven-year-old had succumbed to diphtheria. In May 1900 the *Chicago Daily Tribune* broke the story that John Speicher's seventeen-month-old son died of pneumonia in the Zion Home after a reporter received a tip that Speicher had applied to the city for a burial permit.[14]

Some deaths among Dowie's followers prompted both suspician and legal action. In late July 1899 Annettia Flanders expired in her home under the care of a church elder named DeWitt Holmes and woman named Henrikka Bratsch, one of several female church members Dowie now assigned to attend childbirth cases. At one point during Mrs. Flanders' ordeal her husband, Edward Flanders, sought out a physician's help. When Dr. H. D. Peterson arrived he found the woman "writhing in agony" with a body temperature of 105°. Realizing that the church attendants had done nothing to address her condition, the furious Peterson arranged for Mrs. Flanders to be taken to St. Luke's Hospital, a charity facility in the city's Near South Side; unfortunately, she died there four days later. The physician blamed the death on her attendants' negligence, insisting that had she received competent medical attention sooner her life would have been spared. Peterson was also convinced that "a certain operation had been performed" at some point prior to his arrival. At the coroner's inquest a neighbor reported seeing Bratsch employ unspecified "temporal means" in attending Mrs. Flanders. Although Bratsch initially denied that her ministrations involved anything other than prayer, when pressed by the coroner she admitted she had employed worldly as well as spiritual measures. (The precise nature of Bratsch's actions in attending her patient is unclear. Cook County Coroner's Inquest Records do not include full transcripts of proceedings prior to 1911. The *Journal of the American Medical Association* reported that Bratsch had used scissors to cut the umbilical cord while assisting Mrs. Flanders during childbirth.) The coroner's jury ruled Mrs. Flanders' cause of death to be "peritonitis and puerperal septicemia caused by criminal negligence (malpractice)" and both Bratsch and the church elder Holmes were placed under arrest. A grand jury, however, failed to indict either attendant for criminal acts. Puerperal septicemia, or infection following childbirth, abortion, or miscarriage, was a distressingly common cause of death among women at the end of the nineteenth century and would remain so for several decades into the twentieth. In a report covering the period 1856–1896, the Chicago Board of Health listed infection immediately following childbirth as the cause of death for nearly thirteen percent of all women who died between the ages of twenty and fifty. Perhaps recognizing that deaths due to puerperal septicemia were not uncommon, and unable to ascertain with certainty that the attendants' actions had been the cause of the fatal infection, the grand jury declined to hold them criminally responsible for the woman's death.[15]

Like the Abby Corner case in Boston, the investigation into Annettia Flanders' death confounded the legal boundaries between religious healing and practicing medicine. Asked by reporters to comment on potential charges against the church attendants, Illinois State Board of Health Secretary J. A. Egan asserted that, while Dowie's followers had every right to pray for the sick, they nevertheless were "just as liable for malpractice as any licensed physician" when their earthly ministrations to their patients went wrong. For her part, Bratsch remained confident that the law had no jurisdiction at all over her practices, telling a reporter, "I got my license from God." She herself attributed the woman's death, not to a failure of divine healing, but rather to Edward Flanders' lack of faith. "When he said he was going to call a doctor I nearly cried, because I knew she would die then," Bratsch told the *Tribune*. "God hates medicine." Unlike his wife, Edward Flanders was not a church member and, according to Brastch, he had "made fun of the faith." John Speicher reiterated Bratsch's conviction that Annettia Flanders died because she was removed from God's care. (St. Luke's Hospital had been run by the Episcopal Church since 1865.) "There are lots of lying physicians in the city and they are always giving us trouble," Speicher added, apparently in reference to Dr. Peterson's unwelcome intervention in the case.[16]

Church members' confidence that the law was on their side derived from a new statute signed by Governor John R. Tanner just three months earlier. The Illinois Medical Practice Act of 1899 defined a medical practitioner as anyone "who shall treat or profess to treat, operate on or prescribe for any physical ailment or any physical injury to or deformity of another," and established more stringent educational and licensure requirements for those claiming to practice medicine in the state. The statutory overhaul had come after an intense struggle among the state's regular physicians, who had divided bitterly over the question of whether to force out of business entirely the numerous sectarian practitioners then operating in Illinois, or alternatively, to co-opt them by educating and licensing alternative healers under the regulars' supervision. But, most importantly for Dowie and his associates, the new law specified that its stricter provisions did not apply to "any person who ministers to or treats the sick or suffering by mental or spiritual means, without the use of any drug or material remedy." Caught off guard, the Illinois medical establishment was furious that the religious healing exception had been allowed to slip into the bill, apparently the result of intense lobbying by Chicago-based Christian Scientists. The *Illinois Medical Journal*, the official organ of the Illinois State Medical Society, blamed physicians' lack of professional organization and political unity for the debacle and called for more direct and active involvement by regular doctors in the state's legislative affairs. According to historian Rennie B. Schoepflin, after scoring their initial success in Illinois, Christian Scientists went on to secure exemptions for religious healing in medical practice statutes enacted in twenty-seven more states by the time the nation entered the First World War.[17]

Church members could not yet rest easy, however, for the State Board of Health took action against Henrikka Bratsch for practicing medicine without a license despite the new law's religious exemption. At the trial, Dr. Peterson testified that, upon arriving at the dying woman's bedside, he had noted that "someone had performed the duties of a physician in a bungling way," an assertion that was later supported by the testimony of Annettia Flanders' neighbor. Edward Flanders told the court Bratsch had attempted to relieve his wife's sufferings using "manual treatments" and, when he objected, the attendant had ordered him out of the room; it was at that point that he sought the physician's help. Defending Henrikka Bratsch, attorney Samuel W. Packard (the prestigious—and presumably expensive— Chicago lawyer who now represented Dowie in his myriad legal affairs) brought no rebuttal witnesses, asserting only that Bratsch's case must be dismissed because the Medical Practice Act of 1899 shielded her religious ministrations from state interference. But the court found the attendant guilty, fining her one hundred dollars and court costs. In announcing his ruling, Justice John C. Everett explained that because Bratsch "fell back upon her experience and not upon her faith" in treating Mrs. Flanders, she had crossed a line between offering spiritual support and practicing medicine. Judge Everett's ruling made it clear that secular law could claim jurisdiction when faith healing practices had tangible consequences for the human body. Following the ruling, the Illinois State Board of Health acknowledged that it regarded Bratsch's prosecution as merely the first shot across the bow in a drive to close down Dowie's divine healing operations. "We have been after them a long while," John A. Barnes, the board's counsel told the *Chicago Daily Tribune*. "And I believe that finally we have procured tangible means of bringing certain persistent offenders to justice." Barnes also made it known he intended to revoke the medical license of John Speicher.[18]

Bratsch appealed the ruling in the Illinois Supreme Court but lost her case in February 1902. Later that year, the court determined that the 1899 medical practice act also applied to Joseph V. Gordon, an osteopath and "magnetic" healer. Gordon had appealed his conviction for violating the act by arguing that, because the treatments he proffered involved neither drugs nor surgical appliances, he could not be considered a medical practitioner under the statute's definition. The court, however, disagreed, determining that Gordon's practice involved "knowledge of the location and offices of the various nerves, muscles and joints, the manipulation of those parts and the flexing of the limbs." For the court, various forms of metaphysical healing became the practice of medicine at precisely the point at which the practitioner made contact with the physical body of the patient. Legal regulation of such practices was necessary, the court reasoned, in order to protect the public from "the ignorant and unlearned who hold themselves out as being possessed of peculiar skill in the treatment of disease." In both rulings, the state's highest court legally reinforced the efforts of regular medical doctors to define and enforce what it meant to practice medicine in Illinois.[19]

As the courts forged a path through the new landscape of religious healing and scientific medicine, two more disturbing cases brought divine healing before the courts yet again. In May 1901 a woman named Emma Judd gave birth at home under the care of two church attendants, Henrikka Bratsch and Mary Speicher, the mother of John Speicher. Emma Judd was the wife of Hiram Worthington Judd, recently brought into Dowie's church as the "superintendent" of a new enterprise, the Zion City Land and Investment Association. Sadly, neither the mother nor the baby survived an ordeal made particularly troubling because Emma Judd had suffered convulsions and profuse bleeding from her mouth for a full sixteen hours prior to her death. Despite her prolonged suffering no one attending at Emma Judd's bedside sought medical help, nor did they call the coroner's office when she finally expired. Neighbors, however, saw the body being removed from the home and alerted the police. A physician in the coroner's office then tracked down the remains to an undertaker's establishment where, after examining the body, he determined that Emma Judd had died of a cerebral hemorrhage. Just two days later the same undertaker contacted the coroner about another woman's death, this one occurring in the Zion Home. The undertaker wanted to verify that John Speicher's signature on the death certificate was valid before he took the body to his funeral home. The coroner, John Traeger, ordered the deceased not to be removed from the Zion Home until someone from his office could conduct a postmortem examination. By the time a physician arrived, however, the body had been "spirited away" by church elders, to a different undertaker's establishment located quite a distance away from the South Loop. Furious, Traeger looked into taking possible legal actions against the church elders. He also ordered the exhumation of Emma Judd's remains for further investigation.[20]

At the Judd inquest the evidence presented to the coroner's jury proved to be very grim indeed. Hiram Judd, who had "the appearance of a well-to-do business man," described holding his wife down on their bed as she struggled through her convulsions, placing cloths in her mouth to soak up the blood. Judd explained that church elders had counseled him not to call the coroner's office when his wife finally expired because it might arouse his neighbors' hostilities. He asserted that Emma Judd was a devout follower of Dowie and she had requested prayers but never medical help prior to lapsing into unconsciousness. Following Hiram Judd's testimony several physicians offered professional opinions that the woman's life could have been saved with timely medical intervention. One of them was the noted pathologist Ludvig Hektoen, a student of Christian Fenger who had examined Mrs. Judd's exhumed remains at Cook County Hospital at the request of Coroner Traeger. Originally trained in obstetrics, Hektoen was a pathologist at Cook County Hospital and was also the author of a recent medical school textbook on new techniques of postmortem examination. The pathologist agreed that the cause of death had been cerebral hemorrhage, but added his own finding that the victim had also suffered a hemorrhage of the uterus. He concluded that both bleeds had been caused by Mrs. Judd's excessive straining during prolonged childbirth. Hektoen's examination had revealed she had a condition known as *placenta previa* in which the placenta covered the cervical opening, obstructing the progress of the birth.[21]

John Speicher next explained to jurors that, despite Emma Judd's lengthy ordeal, church members "don't believe in aiding mothers, no matter what the conditions." Taking his own turn on the stand Dowie, who had arrived at the jury room flanked by Zion Guards, described how, upon learning of Emma Judd's difficulties, he had rushed to her bedside and placed his hand upon her chest, whereupon her convulsions immediately subsided. He then left the house "with high hopes of her recovery." Coroner Traeger asked the divine healer if he had made any attempt to ascertain the woman's medical condition, to which Dowie replied, "I am not a physician and I never attempt to act as one." He went on to explain that the church's attendants were "trained nurses [who were] needed to give aid" to women in childbirth. When questioned by Traeger Dowie clarified that by "trained" he meant that he required the attendants to have prior experience assisting with births. Henrikka Bratsch, having learned a lesson from her previous conviction in the Annettia Flanders case, maintained that she had never touched Emma Judd's body at all, leaving the woman entirely under the care of Hiram Judd once the convulsions began. The jury determined the cause of Emma Judd's death to be "cerebral and uterine hemorrhage superinduced by childbirth and complicated by placenta previa." Further, it noted that "if proper medical attendance had been furnished to the said Emma L. Judd she would not have met her death in the manner and form described." Both female birth attendants as well as John Speicher, Hiram Judd, and Dowie himself were placed under arrest. Appearing before the grand jury Ludvig Hektoen chose his words very carefully. He stated that, while he felt certain that medical assistance could have "prolonged life for some hours, and possibly could have saved mother and child," he could not state definitively that Emma Judd would have survived under a physician's care. Perhaps mindful of the degree of medical uncertainty in this case, the grand jury chose not to indict any of the participants. After the hearing one juror told the *Chicago Daily Tribune* that some of his fellow panelists had been uncertain whether religious healers were subject to secular law. The *New York Times* scoffed that the Chicago grand jury proceedings afforded Dowie the opportunity to "pose as a martyr" and predicted the divine healer would now bear the "bravado born of knowing the law does not cover his case."[22]

Incredibly, at the same time he was entangled in the Emma Judd case, Dowie became involved in yet another controversy. On May 5, 1901 a fire broke out in a South Side apartment house, killing seven people and injuring eight more. As the building burned a Dowie follower named Louis Christensen used a rope to lower each of his four children to the sidewalk from the window of their third-floor flat. Unfortunately in the process of the rescue Christensen's youngest child, two-year-old Mabel, received severe burns on her face and arms. Then, before he could help his wife Mary to escape their apartment, she caught fire and, in a panic, jumped to the street below. Barely escaping the terrifying ordeal with their lives, the Christensens sought refuge in the nearby home of the McKee family. When the McKees realized the extent of the injuries sustained by both Mary and Mabel they offered to get medical help but Louis Christensen refused to allow it. But the little girl persisted in crying and tearing at her clothes and the McKees, believing the child to be in intense pain, insisted she receive immediate medical attention, whereupon Christensen abruptly left the premises carrying the baby with him. The McKees then called the police and their ward alderman, who arranged for an ambulance to transport Mary Christensen to the Zion Home as she requested. Sadly, Mrs. Christensen died there ten days later. At the subsequent coroner's inquest several physicians offered opinions that Mary Christensen's injuries, caused by both the fire and her jump from the third floor of the building, had been so severe she was unlikely to have survived even with mainstream medical treatment. The church deacon who had supervised Christensen's care in the Zion Home explained that he had dressed her extensive burns with Vaseline and olive oil and then wrapped them in cloth bandages, a customary form of palliative treatment that did not require specialized expertise. Attendants testified they had been mindful of the need for sanitation, changed the dressings frequently, and kept the room at a warm temperature. They also confirmed that Mrs. Christensen, who stayed conscious throughout her ordeal, had expressed a desire to die but adamantly refused medical attention, not even morphine to ease her extreme pain. The coroner's jury ruled that Mary Christensen died of natural causes that warranted no further legal actions. But it also stated she had not received proper medical attention for her injuries in the Zion Home and censured the "parties in charge" for not seeking it. Finally, jury members recommended that "the proper authorities take steps to prohibit the use of the said house as a Hospital." As he had done previously, city health commissioner Reynolds sent Dowie an application for a hospital license, which of course the divine healer resolutely rejected.[23]

Tragic cases such as those of Annettia Flanders, Emma Judd, and Mary Christensen raised complex and difficult questions about individual conscience and physical suffering. But these women had been adults and presumably fully cognizant of the potentially fatal consequences of eschewing medical assistance when faced with their own extreme trials. Cases involving children proved to be another matter, however, in the court of public opinion as well as under the law; both judged the actions taken by Louis Christensen after the deadly fire in harsh terms. After he had abruptly left the McKee home carrying two-year-old Mabel with him, the Chicago police found Mr. Christensen walking on the street and attempted to wrest the burned child from his arms by force. When the distraught father resisted, an officer charged him with disorderly conduct and placed him under arrest. Because Mabel was deemed to be a victim of medical neglect, an agent of the Illinois Humane Society was alerted to her case. Either unaware of, or merely ignoring, Christensen's religious convictions the society's agent asserted his own quasi-legal authority and took Mabel to a physician for treatment of her burns. The baby resided briefly at the doctor's own home until a judge was able to locate nearby relatives, despite the fact that Christensen had been released on bail and presumably able to care for his daughter. In placing the child in the family member's custody, the court stipulated that Mabel would be returned to her father only after she had recovered from her injuries. Predictably, Dowie reacted with outrage to the court's actions "We will not suffer our children to be taken out of our hands," he thundered in the pages of *Leaves of Healing*. "Zion's first work is to care for her children." He took the opportunity to once again rail against laws that forced parents to obtain medical care for children over their religious objections. He also took the opportunity to renew his call against the use of antitoxin, once again asserting the sinfulness of the new serum therapy. Dowie claimed that, while children being treated with antitoxin in Chicago had been dying in droves, "our children have been kept, and are alive." The divine healer then suggested he would assist parents who, like Louis Christensen, stood fast in their faith and resisted authorities' attempts to force mainstream medicine on children. "We are prepared to fight in open court the question as to whether healing through faith in Jesus Christ is not better than drugs or doctors," he asserted. Dowie dared his nemesis, the Chicago city health commission Arthur Reynolds, to publicly debate him on the topic of divine healing versus science.[24]

Soon, however, John Alexander Dowie had much higher matters to attend to than the machinations of his earthly enemies. Within the year the General Overseer of the Christian Catholic Church was busy moving his followers to a new community, Zion City, located fifty miles outside of Chicago in Lake County, Illinois. The new site placed the church far from the relentless pursuit of physicians in the offices of the Chicago city health commissioner and the Cook County coroner. The faithful bought shares in the new enterprise at one hundred dollars apiece through the Zion Land and Investment Association. Then, in June 1901, Dowie made the startling revelation that he was a prophet, Elijah the Restorer. "I have come to proclaim theocracy pure and simple," he declared before a capacity crowd in the Chicago Auditorium. "I will never rest till all other forms of government have been driven from the earth."[25]

Although Dowie relocated his family to Zion City, his twenty-three-year-old daughter Esther retained her own residence in the Zion Home, finding the downtown location more convenient as she pursued her studies at the University of Chicago. On the morning of May 16, 1902, Esther readied herself for the day ahead. She placed her curling iron on a spirit lamp, a small appliance that created heat by burning alcohol. Somehow, Esther upset the lamp and her dressing gown caught fire. Zion Home residents heard her screams and came to her aid, but tragically the young woman sustained severe burns over three-quarters of her body. John Speicher carefully washed and dressed the extensive wounds. Dowie was summoned by telephone and, immediately upon his arrival, prayed at Esther's bedside. After several hours, however, it became clear that the young woman's condition was deteriorating rapidly and the situation was indeed most dire. At that point, the divine healer and holy warrior took an extraordinary step. He sent Speicher to retrieve A. W. Campbell, a regular medical doctor whose practice was located nearby to the Zion Home. It was the desperate, and very human, act of a father attempting to save the life of his beloved only daughter. Sadly, Esther Dowie died that evening.[26]

# NOTES

1. John Alexander Dowie, *Zion's Holy War Against the Hosts of Hell in Chicago* (Chicago: Zion Publishing House, 1900), 19, 148; Gordon Lindsay, editor, *The Sermons of John Alexander Dowie* (Shreveport, LA: Voice of Healing Publishing, n.d.), 25; Edna Sheldrake, editor, *The Personal Letters of John Alexander Dowie* (Zion City, IL: Wilbur Glenn Voliva, 1912), 314–318; "Baffled by No Disease," *Chicago Daily Tribune* (October 3, 1890): 1. On Dowie's extraordinary life, see Philip L. Cook, *Zion City, Illinois* (Syracuse University Press, 1996); Alden H. Heath, "Apostle in Zion," *Journal of the Illinois State Historical Society*, Volume 70, Number 2 (May 1977): 98–113; Gordon Lindsey, *John Alexander Dowie: A Life Story of Trials, Tragedies and Triumphs* (Shreveport, LA: Voice of Healing Publishing, 1951); Grant Wacker, "Marching to Zion: Religion in a Modern Utopian Community," *Church History*, Volume 54, Number 4 (December 1985): 496–511; Zion Historical Society, *Zion* (Charleston, SC: Arcadia Publishing, 2007).

2. *Leaves of Healing*, Volume 1, Number 1 (August 31, 1894): 2, 14–16; *Leaves of Healing*, Volume 3, Number 30 (May 22, 1897): 471; "Preached in a Big Tent," *Chicago Daily Tribune* (July 28, 1890): 5.

3. *Leaves of Healing*, Volume 3, Number 24 (April 10, 1897): 381; "All Draw Heavily: Report of Controller Ackerman to Council," *Chicago Daily Tribune* (November 1, 1894): 5; John Alexander Dowie, *Doctors, Drugs, and Devils* (Zion City, IL: Zion Publishing House, 1901), 18.

4. Joseph W. Williams, *Spirit Cure: A History of Pentecostal Healing* (New York: Oxford University Press, 2013); Heather D. Curtis, *Faith in the Great Physician: Suffering and Divine Healing in American Culture, 1860–1900* (Baltimore: Johns Hopkins University Press, 2007); David Edwin Harrell Jr., "Divine Healing in Modern American Protestantism," in Norman Gevitz, editor, *Other Healers: Unorthodox Medicine in America* (Baltimore: Johns Hopkins University Press, 1988), 215–227; Walter J. Hollenweger, *The Pentecostals* (Minneapolis: Augsburg Press, 1972).

5. Timothy E. W. Gloege, "Faith Healing, Medical Regulation, and Public Religion in Progressive Era Chicago," *Religion and American Culture: A Journal of Interpretation*, Volume 23, Number 2 (Summer 2013): 185–231; Ronald L. Numbers, *Prophetess of Health: A Study of Ellen G. White*. Third edition (Grand Rapids, MI: William B. Eerdmans Publishing Company, 2008); Brian C. Wilson, *Dr. John Harvey Kellogg and the Religion of Biologic Living* (Bloomington: Indiana University Press, 2014); Cook, *Zion City, Illinois*, 57–58, 172; Robert C. Fuller, *The Body of Faith: A Biological History of Religion in America* (Chicago: University of Chicago Press, 2013), 111; Shirley Nelson, *Fair, Clear, and Terrible: The Story of Shiloh* (Eugene, OR: Wipf and Stock, 2009), 151–152.

6. "Dowie Threatens His Foes," *Chicago Daily Tribune* (November 6, 1899): 3; "Run Out of Town," *Chicago Daily Tribune* (October 28, 1899): 1; "Dowie Mobbed in Indiana," *New York Times* (October 29, 1899): 12. The numerous contemporary accounts of anti-Dowie demonstrations include: "Riot at Dowie Lecture," *Chicago Daily Tribune* (October 19, 1899): 1; "Dowie Tours the City," *Chicago Daily Tribune* (October 23, 1899); "Cat Calls for Zionist Dowie," *New York Times* (October 17, 1900): 6; "Rioting at Dowie Meeting," *New York Times* (October 24, 1900): 7; "Zion Guards in Riot," *Chicago Record-Herald* (July 11, 1901); "Dowieites to Keep Peace in Evanston," *Chicago Record-Herald* (July 11, 1901); "Hose Played on Zionists by Evanston Firemen," *New York Times* (July 11, 1901): 1. Historian Michael Sappol points out that riots by medical students were not unknown in the nineteenth century, particularly in response to legal prohibitions on the procuring of cadavers by medical schools. *A Traffic of Dead Bodies: Anatomy and Embodied Social Identity in Nineteenth-Century America* (Princeton: Princeton University Press, 2002).

7. "Brother Tries to Get Boy from Zion," *Chicago Daily Tribune* (July 22, 1903): 3. Rolvix Harlan leveled his critique of the divine healer in *John Alexander Dowie and the Christian Catholic Apostolic Church* (Evansville, WI: Press of Robert M. Antes, 1906), 117. On divine healing communities that emerged outside of Chicago, see James Opp, *The Lord for the Body: Religion, Medicine, and Protestant Faith Healing in Canada, 1880–1930* (Montreal: McGill-Queen's University Press), 103–114.

8. Dowie, *Zion's Holy War*, 119; Dowie, *Doctors, Drugs, and Devils*, 30; Heath, "Apostle in Zion," 108; *Leaves of Healing*, Volume 1, Number 17 (January 11, 1895): 257–263; "Divine Healing the Antidote to Christian Science, Falsely So-Called," *Leaves of Healing*, Volume 1, Number 4 (September 21, 1894): 68.

9. Thomas Bonner, *Medicine in Chicago, 1850–1950*. Second edition (Urbana: University of Illinois Press, 1991); George W. Webster, "Medical Legislation Concerning Medical Education in Illinois," *Illinois Medical Journal*, Volume XXI, Number 3 (March 1912): 332–339. The Illinois State Board of Health was among the most active state societies in pressing for higher standards of medical education. Richard Harrison Shryock, *Medical Licensing in America, 1650–1965* (Baltimore: Johns Hopkins University Press, 1967), 53–55. On the fierce competition between regular and sectarian practitioners at the turn of the twentieth century, see Michael H. Cohen, *Complementary & Alternative Medicine: Legal Boundaries and Regulatory Perspectives* (Baltimore: Johns Hopkins University Press, 1995); James C. Whorton, *Nature Cures: The History of Alternative Medicine in America* (New York: Oxford University Press, 2002); Owen Whooley, *Knowledge in the Time of Cholera: The Struggle over American*

*Medicine in the Nineteenth Century* (Chicago: University of Chicago Press, 2013); Susan E. Cayleff, *Nature's Path: A History of Naturopathic Healing in America* (Baltimore: Johns Hopkins University Press, 2016). On medical licensing as a political strategy used by regular practitioners to eliminate their competition, see Paul Starr, *The Social Transformation of American Medicine* (New York: Basic Books); David A. Johnson and Humayn J. Chaudhry, editors, *Medical Licensing and Discipline in America: A History of the Federation of State Medical Boards* (Lanham, MD: Lexington Books, 2012); James C. Mohr, *Licensed to Practice: The Supreme Court Defines the American Medical Profession* (Baltimore: Johns Hopkins University Press, 2013).

10. On the Chicago city health commissioner, see Arthur R. Reynolds Reynolds, "Reminiscences of Ten Years as Commissioner of Health in Chicago, and Suggestions for the Future," *California State Journal of Medicine*, Volume VII, Number 6: 218–221; Bonner, *Medicine in Chicago*, 205–206. Dowie's arrest in Melbourne is described in Sheldrake, *The Personal Letters of John Alexander Dowie*, 322. On his legal troubles in Chicago in 1895, see "Faith-Healer Dowie Arrested," *Chicago Daily Tribune* (January 6, 1895): 1; "Visit Dowie's Homes," *Chicago Daily Tribune* (January 8, 1895): 12; "Dowie's Race Is Nearly Run," *Chicago Daily Tribune* (January 9, 1895): 8; "To Protect the Sick," *Chicago Daily Tribune* (January 13, 1895): 10; "Dowie Roasts His Persecutors," *Chicago Daily Tribune* (June 24, 1895): 3; "Dowie Jury Reports Disagreement," *Chicago Daily Tribune* (June 26, 1895): 8; "Dowie's Jury Under Suspicion," *Chicago Daily Tribune* (June 27, 1895): 8; "Drugs of No Use Now," *Chicago Daily Tribune* (July 3, 1895): 12; "Dowie Invites Contagious Disease," *Chicago Daily Tribune* (July 12, 1895): 8; "Dowie Says He Is Not a Nuisance," *Chicago Daily Tribune* (July 13, 1895): 13; "John Alexander Dowie's Case," *Chicago Daily Tribune* (July 16, 1895): 6; "One Hundred Dollar Fine for Dowie," *Chicago Daily Tribune* (July 19, 1895): 1; "Another Jury Finds Dowie Guilty," *Chicago Daily Tribune* (August 3, 1895): 4; "What Is a Hospital?" *Chicago Daily Tribune* (August 9, 1895): 1; "Leo Maguire et al. v. John Alexander Dowie," *Leaves of Healing*, Volume 1, Number 46 (August 16, 1895): 725; "'Dr' Dowie's Day in Court," *Chicago Daily Tribune* (August 17, 1895): 5.

11. *Leaves of Healing*, Volume 1, Number 1 (August 31, 1894): 9–13. Dowie printed a partial transcript of the proceedings in his fraud case in issues of *Leaves of Healing*, Volume 1, Number 19 (January 25, 1895): 293–301; Volume 1, Number 20 (February 2, 1895): 309; Volume 1, Number 22 (February 15, 1895): 337; "Dowie in Trouble Again," *Chicago Daily Tribune* (October 4, 1896): 7. See also: "'Dr.' Dowie's Case Again," *Chicago Daily Tribune* (January 16, 1895): 8; "Dowie on the Stand for Himself,"

*Chicago Daily Tribune* (January 23, 1895): 9; "'Divine Healer' Dowie Fined $100," *Chicago Daily Tribune* (February 3, 1895): 6. The case of the itinerant medicine seller is *State v. Blue Mountain Joe*, 129 Ill. 370, 1889.

12. On Christian Fenger's influence on Chicago medical education, see Bonner, *Medicine in Chicago*, 85–86; David J. Davis, editor, *The History of Medical Practice in Illinois*, Volume II, 1850–1900 (Chicago: Illinois State Medical Society, 1955), 208–209; Arthur E. Hertzler, *The Horse and Buggy Doctor* (New York: Harper and Brothers, 1938), 47–50. The plan for modernizing the Cook County Coroner's Office is described in "May Be End to Coroner's Work," *Chicago Daily Tribune* (October 15, 1900): 1. The historical transition from coroner's juries to medical examiners' offices is discussed in Katherine D. Watson, *Forensic Medicine in Western Society: A History* (New York: Routledge, 2011).

13. "He Dies at Dowie's," *Chicago Daily Tribune* (June 24, 1894): 11; "Funeral of Professor Kellogg," *Chicago Daily Tribune* (June 27, 1894): 2. "Drugs of No Use Now," *Chicago Daily Tribune* (July 3, 1895): 12; "Dies in Dowie's Den," *Chicago Daily Tribune* (July 2, 1895).

14. "Victim of a Faith," *Chicago Daily Tribune* (February 27, 1899); "Coroners Blame Dowie Plan," *Chicago Daily Tribune* (October 20, 1899): 1; "Boy Clings to Belief in Divine Healing and Death Results," *Chicago Daily Tribune* (June 24, 1900): 8; "Ollie Kendall Prefers Dying in Dowie Church to Living by Medicines," *Chicago Daily Tribune* (September 16, 1900): 1; "Girl Dies in Dowie Zion," *Chicago Daily Tribune* (October 26, 1900): 1; "Dies During 'Zion' Cure," *Chicago Daily Tribune* (December 26, 1899): 1; "Die Despite Dowie Prayers," *Chicago Daily Tribune* (March 2, 1900): 1; "Autopsy on a Dowie Patient," *Chicago Daily Tribune* (March 24, 1900): 7; "Two Die in Dowie's House," *Chicago Daily Tribune* (May 20, 1900): 1.

15. Inquest on Annettia Flanders, *Cook County Medical Examiner's Reports*, No. 16613, July 28 and August 8, 1899 (Illinois Regional Archives Depository, Northeastern Illinois University, Chicago, IL); "D. C. Holmes and Mrs. Bratsch Free," *Chicago Daily Tribune* (September 26, 1899): 12; "Construction of Illinois Law and Dowie Treatment," *Journal of the American Medical Association*, Volume XXXIII, Number 15 (October 7, 1899): 929–930. On St. Luke's Hospital, see Bonner, *Medicine in Chicago*, 152–153. On puerperal septicemia as a cause of death in Chicago, see Bonner, *Medicine in Chicago*, 22–31.

16. "She Had Faith but Dies," *Chicago Daily Tribune* (July 29, 1899): 1; "Move in Flanders Case," *Chicago Daily Tribune* (July 30, 1899): 5; "Dowie People Use Placards," *Chicago Daily Tribune* (August 8, 1899): 12; "Invoke Law on Dowie," *Chicago Daily Tribune* (August 15, 1899): 10. In its own coverage of the case the *New York Times* initially misidentified

the practitioners as Christian Scientists. "Christian Scientists Held," *New York Times* (August 9, 1899): 2.

17. Illinois State Board of Health, *Report on Medical Education and Official Register of Legally Qualified Physicians* (Springfield: Illinois State Register, 1903): xvii; J. W. Pettit, "The Present Law," *Illinois Medical Journal*, Volume XLIX, Number 10 (April 1900): 467–472; Rennie B. Schoepflin, *Christian Science on Trial: Religious Healing in America* (Baltimore: Johns Hopkins University Press, 2003), 164.

18. "To Sift 'Divine Healing," *Chicago Daily Tribune* (July 31, 1899): 12; "Jail for Faith Healers," *Chicago Daily Tribune* (August 9, 1899): 12. "Faith Healing," *The Illinois Medical Journal*, Volume XLIX, Number 3 (September 1899): 130–132; "A Conviction Under the New Medical Practice Act," *The Illinois Medical Journal*, Volume XLIX, Number 4 (October 1899): 174–176. Dowie's attorney Samuel Packard is described in John McAuley Palmer, editor, *The Bench and Bar of Illinois: Historical and Reminiscent*, Volume 2 (Chicago: The Lewis Publishing Company, 1899), 1224–1226. John C. Everett is listed as a Justice of the Peace for South Chicago in *The Chicago Daily News Almanac and Year Book* (Chicago: Chicago Daily News Company, 1902), 391.

19. *Henrikka Bratsch v. The People*, 195 Ill. 165 (February 21, 1902); *People of the State of Illinois v. Joseph P. Gordon* 194 Ill. 560 (February 21, 1902). On osteopathy and magnetic healing, see Norman Gevitz, *The DOs: Osteopathic Medicine in America*. Second edition (Baltimore: Johns Hopkins University Press, 2004).

20. "Two Die While 'Dr' Dowie Prays," *Chicago Daily Tribune* (May 14, 1901): 1; "Police Called to Dowie Bank," *Chicago Daily Tribune* (May 19, 1901): 3.

21. Inquest on Emma L. Judd, *Cook County Medical Examiner's Reports*, No. 20660, May 13, 16, and 23, 1901. Illinois Regional Archives Depository, Northeastern Illinois University, Chicago, Illinois. On Ludvig Hektoen, see Bonner, *Medicine in Chicago*, 90–92.

22. "Law Hits Zion, Dowie Is Held," *Chicago Daily Tribune* (May 2, 1901); 1; "Dowie Pictures a Death Scene," *Chicago Daily Tribune* (May 17, 1901): 1; "New Move Against Dowie," *Chicago Record-Herald* (May 21, 1901); "Dowie in New Danger," *Chicago Daily Herald* (May 23, 1901); "Warrant Out for J. A. Dowie," *New York Times* (May 24, 1901): 2; "More Trouble for Dowie," *Chicago Record-Herald* (May 25, 1901); "Dowie in Bonds, Wrath on Zion," *Chicago Daily Tribune* (May 25, 1901): 3; "Law's Batteries Open on Dowie," *Chicago Daily Tribune* (May 28, 1901): 1; "Dowie Asks Police Guard," *Chicago Daily Tribune* (May 30, 1901): 2; "Legal Dilemma Menaces Dowie," *Chicago Daily Tribune* (May 29, 1901): 3; "Dowie Waits His Fate," *Chicago Record-Herald* (May 30, 1901); "Grand

Jury Frees Dowie," *Chicago Daily Tribune* (June 2, 1901): 5; "To Make Chicago Clean," *New York Times* (June 2, 1901): 20.

23. "Seven Perish in Blazing House," *Chicago Daily Tribune* (May 6, 1901): 1; "Features and Actors in the Fire Horror at South Chicago," *Chicago Daily Tribune* (May 6, 1901): 2; "Victim of Fire, Then of Dowie," *Chicago Daily Tribune* (May 16, 1901): 1; "Dowieites Remain Loyal," *Chicago Daily Herald* (May 22, 1901); "Say Zion Uses Aid to Prayer," *Chicago Daily Tribune* (May 22, 1901): 1; Inquest on Mary Louisa Christensen, *Cook County Medical Examiner's Reports*, No. 20669, May 16, 21, and 24, 1901. Illinois Regional Archives Depository, Northeastern Illinois University, Chicago, Illinois.

24. "Hide Baby from Zion Treatment," *Chicago Daily Tribune* (May 7, 1901): 3; "Dispute About a Child," *New York Times* (May 7, 1901): 2; *Leaves of Healing*, Volume IX, Number 9 (June 22, 1901): 272; "Dowie Utters Defiance," *Chicago Record Herald* (June 17, 1901).

25. "I Am Elijah—Dowie," *Chicago Record-Herald* (June 3, 1901); "Dowie Utters Defiance," *Chicago Record Herald* (June 17, 1901); "Esther Dowie Dead," *New York Times* (May 16, 1902): 2; "Dowie Girl Dead, Funeral at Zion," *Chicago Daily Tribune* (May 16, 1902): 3.

26. Dowie's graphically detailed account of Esther's death, in which he included a transcript of the coroner's inquest, is "Story of the Fatal Injury and Triumphant Departure," *Leaves of Healing*, Volume XI, Number 4 (May 17, 1902): 107–115.

# CHAPTER 7

# Children's Medical Care in the Courts

We place no limitations upon the power of the mind over the body, the power
of faith to dispel disease, or the power of the Supreme Being to heal the sick.
We merely declare the law as given us by the legislature.

In October 1903 New York's highest court sustained a father's criminal
conviction for refusing to seek medical assistance for his dying child. Two
years earlier J. Luther Pierson's sixteen-month-old adopted daughter had
succumbed to pneumonia after being ill for several weeks with pertussis, or
whooping cough. At his trial Pierson, a railroad engineer from White Plains,
explained his adherence to John Alexander Dowie's teaching that sickness
came from the devil and thus only God could cure it; he also believed his
own prayers could serve as a conduit for divine healing power. While he
had not anticipated her death, Pierson acknowledged he had been aware
the child was gravely ill for a period of at least forty-eight hours before she
expired. Nevertheless, he remained adamant in his faith, telling the court he
had not—and would never–seek a physician's aid, no matter how serious a
child's illness might appear. He believed his daughter had died, not because
she lacked medical attention, but rather because his own faith in divine
healing had not been strong enough. The court instructed jury members
that, while they could not evaluate the validity of Pierson's religious beliefs,

© The Author(s) 2019
L. Curry, *Religion, Law, and the Medical Neglect
of Children in the United States, 1870–2000,*
Palgrave Studies in the History of Childhood,
https://doi.org/10.1007/978-3-030-24689-1_7

they *could* consider his awareness of the little girl's distressed physical state at the time he refused to seek medical assistance for her. The question to deliberate, according to the court, was whether this father had intentionally refused "to call in a physician or give [the child] such medicines as the science of the age would say [to be] proper." The jury found Pierson guilty and the court fined him the considerable sum of five hundred dollars, a penalty which he refused to pay, whereupon the court sentenced him to a jail term of five hundred days. (In a sad twist, the *Christian Advocate* reported that Pierson's infant son also died of pneumonia, just one day after the father began his jail sentence.) The trial received widespread newspaper coverage outside of Westchester County. The *New York Times* noted the outcome with approval, remarking that the "White Plains jury is to be congratulated on the intelligence of its jurymen." Dowie's nemesis the *Chicago Daily Tribune* was equally pleased with the trial's result, declaring it definitive proof that "a sick child has its rights."[1]

Such celebrations in the press proved to be premature, however. A New York appeals court reversed the trial court's judgment, finding that the "science of the age" was not in fact the appropriate standard for assessing Pierson's culpability in his daughter's death. The correct measure, according to Judge Willard Bartlett, was whether the father's actions reflected "the conduct of an ordinarily prudent person." Pierson had been convicted under an 1881 revision to the New York penal code making it a misdemeanor for an adult to place a child "in such a situation that its life may be endangered or its health be likely to be injured." Like a number of states, New York had sought to both expand and clarify the definition of child neglect, an effort that augmented traditional concerns about preserving moral order in the community with statutes reflecting new standards for children's physical care informed by medical science, especially the emerging fields of bacteriology and pediatrics. While the law could be construed to require the provision of medical attendance under certain circumstances, Judge Bartlett reasoned, it did not mandate the services of professional medical practitioners in every instance when a child fell ill. To be sure, a very long tradition of household nursing, aided by folk wisdom and popular domestic advice manuals, attested to parents' central role in caring for their children without the interventions of physicians. If the law did not mandate medical assistance in every case of illness or injury, and an "ordinarily prudent person" might very well care for an ailing child without a physician's aid, then the jury could not find a violation in this father's actions. Pierson's criminal conviction was therefore vacated and a new trial ordered.[2]

Judge Bartlett's colleague William W. Goodrich strongly disagreed with this particular rendering of the case. For Goodrich, the key point was that Pierson had not sought aid from an alternative medical practitioner (a homeopathic physician, for example) during his daughter's illness, nor had he consulted any of the numerous published treatises on domestic health care that were widely available to parents. Rather, he had stated plainly that he would not have sought *any* form medical attendance for his daughter other than his own prayers. In a lengthy dissent Goodrich cited the trial testimony of two physicians in the Westchester County coroner's office who had found the child to be "pretty well emaciated" at the time of her death. (Pierson had testified that the baby had been able to take milk but apparently she had eaten little else.) Further, the compromised state of the child's body at the time of her death led the physicians to conclude she had endured "considerable suffering" during her extended illness. Pertussis is an infectious bacterial disease that, like diphtheria, claimed the lives of thousands of young children in the United States at the turn of the twentieth century. While no therapeutic intervention parallel to diphtheria antitoxin existed in 1901, regular medical practitioners did advise parents on various prophylactic measures to ease sufferers' symptoms. A recently published article in the *Journal of the American Medical Association*, for example, noted the effectiveness of Joseph O'Dwyer's specialized tubes in easing the breathing of children suffering from whooping cough. Judge Goodrich argued that, given the baby's age and the protracted nature of the illness, pneumonia posed a serious threat to the child's life and, what is more, Pierson could have known the severity of this risk. By refusing to seek any medical help at all in light of her observable, severely distressed, physical condition, Goodrich reasoned, Pierson had in fact placed his daughter in circumstances that endangered her health and life. Therefore his conduct was nothing less than "a plain refusal to obey the law" as it was expressly written.[3]

Seven months later, J. Luther Pierson's case took yet another twist at New York's highest court where Judge Albert Haight reversed the appellate court ruling and affirmed the trial judge's original instruction to the jury. New York law assigned parents the duty to maintain and preserve the life of their child, Haight wrote for a unanimous court, including an obligation to obtain medical assistance when circumstances required it. For Haight, defining the term "medical assistance" was the key to determining the law's intent. For insight he drew upon the state's medical licensing act which, in 1880, had expressly limited the practice of medicine to those who were duly qualified by virtue of their specialized education and training as delineated in the statute's provisions. Thus, he reasoned, when it revised the penal code the following year, the legislature had intended "medical assistance" to mean taking measures that comported with what the "science of the age" would deem appropriate given a child's physical condition. It was incumbent upon parents, Haight's reasoning suggested, to monitor their children's physical states and to take appropriate actions, including procuring the services of medical professionals when they were required. As precedent Haight cited *Cowley v. New York*, an 1881 case in which the superintendent of a charitable institution had appealed his conviction under the same law that Pierson had been convicted of violating. In that case a jury had heard a physician's testimony describing the extremely emaciated state of a young inmate of the institution; in a novel move, the court also allowed several photographs of the little boy to be admitted as evidence of the superintendent's neglect. The jury found that Edward Cowley violated the law because he failed to provide "proper and sufficient medicine and medical attendance when [the] child was sick, diseased, and ailing." Apparently moved by the photographic evidence, the appeals court went even further, noting that the boy's physical appearance differed so very markedly from that of a healthy child his urgent need for medical care would have been obvious to anyone who merely looked at him. (The court also affirmed that photographs were "products of a scientific process" and thus acceptable as forensic evidence at trial.) Pierson, of course, did not cause the illness that took his daughter's life. Nevertheless, like Cowley, he had been fully aware of a child's deteriorating physical state and therefore his refusal to seek medical help constituted a willful act that endangered her life—in violation of New York's child endangerment law. In affirming Pierson's conviction, Justice Haight underlined the state's authority to intercede on behalf of suffering children when adults failed in their responsibilities toward them. "The law of nature, as well as the common law, devolves upon the parents the duty of caring for our young in sickness and in health, and in doing whatever may be necessary for their care, maintenance and preservation, including medical assistance if necessary," he wrote. "An omission to do this is a public wrong which the state, under its police powers, may prevent." For this court, protecting children's bodies represented a core function of the law, even if it meant interfering in parents' private decisions in caring for them.[4]

At the beginning of the twentieth century, the legal odyssey taken by J. Luther Pierson's case reflected a larger struggle by American courts to redefine adults' duties following preceding decades' heightened attention to children's physical welfare. Historians have noted courts' increased willingness to assert state jurisdiction in matters such as injuries to child industrial workers and sexual violence perpetrated against minors.[5] The common law legal doctrine known as *parens patriae* asserted the power of the state to protect individuals who were unable to care for themselves. Prior to 1800, however, courts had generally deferred to the authority of parents—particularly of fathers—in matters pertaining to the children living in their own households, among whom could be counted indentured servants, apprentices, and slaves as well as biological offspring. Anglo-American legal traditions, however, privileged fathers' vested rights to obedience, labor, and support rather than concerns for children's physical well-being. As Mark E. Brandon has observed, the common law granted a father "broad discretion as to whether and how to maintain his children." In most cases, the obligation extended only to "necessaries," or those things required to sustain a child's life, rather than to "superfluities," or provisions that exceeded, in either quantity or quality, the most basic requirements for survival. Apprenticeship contracts, for example, typically obligated masters to provide food and clothing to the young charges residing in their households, but such provisions need only be "suitable for an apprentice"—enough to meet the basic survival needs of a child who occupied that particular social station. Legal requirements concerning children's maintenance were not intended to *improve* the conditions into which they had been born, but rather to prepare children to assume their rightful places within a local community hierarchy, thereby perpetuating moral order and social stability. Thus the distinctions to be made between the categories of "necessaries" and "superfluities" varied in accordance with a minor's age, sex, race, and legal status.[6]

Over the course of the nineteenth century, the legal landscape of family relations changed dramatically in the United States as courts increasingly considered children's specialized requirements for physical care. Judges began awarding custody to mothers rather than fathers, for example, particularly in cases involving very young children deemed to be of "tender years" and thus requiring a more intensive degree of nurturing. State courts began holding parents to higher standards in providing for their children's physical needs. In 1870 James Schouler published an influential treatise, *The Law of Domestic Relations*, in which he cited "medical attendance" along with "food, lodging, clothes, and education" among the "five leading elements in the doctrine of the infant's necessaries." For this Massachusetts jurist, medical attendance fell squarely under the category of "necessity" for maintaining the health and life of a child, and the doctrine of *parens patriae* empowered the state to enforce parents' duties to provide for a physician's services when needed.[7]

Schouler's substitution of the modern term "medical attendance" for the archaic term "physick" reflected a professionalization of medical practice evolving in tandem with the emergence of a new legal calculus for determining parental responsibilities. But, even as medical attendance came to be regarded as an obligation in caring for children, delineating a precise meaning for the term itself was no straightforward task. Despite the growing dominance of regular physicians in medicine, a variety of sectarian practitioners, along with various professionals such as midwives, nurses, and pharmacists, remained active participants in the health care universe to which parents had access in the late nineteenth century. The emergence of several new healing religions, most notably Christian Science and the Christian Catholic Church, further complicated the picture. As we have seen, their growing numbers challenged the legal boundaries between religious belief and medical practice. Both Mary Baker Eddy and John Alexander Dowie insisted that constitutional protections for religious freedom exempted their healing activities from interference by secular law. Many jurists, however, were less certain. The foundation for this doubt was established in two separate cases that came before the United State Supreme Court eleven years apart. First, in an often-cited opinion rendered in 1878, the Court upheld the constitutionality of Congress's legal prohibition on polygamy, a practice associated with members of the Church of Jesus Christ of Latter-Day Saints who were then residing in the federal Utah Territory. "Laws are made for the government of actions," Chief Justice Morrison Waite had written for a unanimous court, "and while they cannot interfere with mere religious belief and opinions, they may with practices." In *Reynolds v. United States*, therefore, the nation's high court opened the door to the possibility of governmental entities placing restrictions on the healing activities of religious organizations.[8]

The second opinion was rendered in 1889 when the Court addressed the question of whether individual states could expand their police powers to regulate, or even prohibit, the services of health care practitioners who had been trained in particular schools. In *Dent v. West Virginia* the court affirmed a state's power to define for itself what it meant to practice medicine. The Court rejected a challenge from a healer of the botanical school known as "eclectic" medicine who had been denied a license to practice in that state. Dent claimed that West Virginia's law represented an infringement upon his right to continue plying the vocation he had practiced for ten years prior to the law's passage in 1881. But Justice Stephen J. Field's opinion strongly endorsed the idea that states did in fact possess sufficient powers to require specialized education and training of those to whom it awarded certification:

> No one has a right to practice medicine without having the necessary qualifications of learning and skill; and the statute only requires that whoever assumes, by offering to the community his services as a physician, that he possesses such learning and skill, shall present evidence of it by a certificate or license from a body designated by the state as competent to judge of his qualifications.

A noteworthy dimension of Justice Field's brief opinion is his view of scientific medicine. For Field, a license to practice medicine signaled to the public that a given medical attendant possessed the requisite knowledge and skill to successfully treat cases of illness and injury. In essence, licensure substituted the state's judgment for the patient's, a necessary change given that, by the late nineteenth century, medicine had become complex enough that a practitioner's competency and expertise were difficult for the average person to discern. Excluding the non-qualified from medical practice therefore fell within the state's police powers to protect the public's health and safety. Interestingly, the justice ventured a bit further, asserting that the state may also "call for further conditions as new modes of treating disease are discovered… or a more accurate knowledge is acquired of the human system and of the agencies by which it is affected." Field's construction tacitly acknowledged that those who professed to practice medicine must keep abreast of the science of the age and, what is more, that the state may compel them to do so in order to maintain certification. As an eclectic, Dent was a sectarian rather than a religious practitioner. Nevertheless, the Court's opinion in his case hinted at the dilemma of reconciling the practice of scientific medicine as it had evolved by the late nineteenth century with newly established healing religions predicated on universal and unchanging metaphysical truths, as both Eddy and Dowie taught.[9]

In 1894 Nebraska's Supreme Court held that a law requiring state certification for all those who "profess to heal, or prescribe for or otherwise treat, any physical or mental ailment" had been appropriately extended to practitioners of Christian Science by a lower court. Four years later, however, the Rhode Island Supreme Court drew the line differently, holding that the state's licensing law applied only to medical practice as "ordinarily and popularly understood"—a meaning that did not include "simply praying" for the patient's recovery nor "teaching that disease will disappear," as per Mary Baker Eddy's teachings. A corollary dilemma for the courts was how to determine legal penalties when religious healers' ministrations went wrong. A key precedent had been set early in the century when, in 1809, a Massachusetts jury had refused to convict Samuel Thomson, the founder of the botanical sect known as Thomsonianism, of manslaughter in the death of a patient. The judge in the case had instructed the jury that there could be no crime if Thomson had not acted recklessly or with the intent to cause harm when he treated his patient, who had voluntarily submitted to his care, according to his own healing system. Ninety years later courts continued to grapple with the thorny issue of imposing legal liabilities upon alternative healers, including religious ones. In 1899 New York lawyer William A. Purrington, an outspoken critic of Christian Science, lamented the notion that religious healers' ignorance of scientific medicine could continue to shield them from penalties as America entered the twentieth century. "There is no reason why unqualified persons should be allowed to pretend to cure disease, by their pretenses deprive the sick of the benefits of science, and yet escape the just consequences of their imposture," he insisted. In the previous year a court in Milwaukee, Wisconsin convicted two Christian Science healers of practicing medicine without a license following the death of an eleven-year-old girl from diphtheria. After hearing testimony in which the healers described their interactions with the ailing child over a period of twelve hours, Judge N. B. Neelson rejected the defenses' claim that their ministrations were solely religious in character and thus exempt from regulation by the state. While he affirmed the "perfect freedom" of Christian Scientists to "hold and teach their doctrine," the fact that these practitioners had held themselves out as "able to heal physical ailments" made them subject to state laws requiring the "competent knowledge of those branches of true science" that was necessary to effect cures. In 1904, however, the New Hampshire supreme court took a different view, refusing to award damages to a woman who had sued a Christian Science practitioner on the grounds that his ineffective ministrations had delayed the recovery she would have enjoyed had she been treated by a regular physician.[10]

The ambiguous and confusing case law had critical implications for parents. If the courts did not deem religious healers to be legitimate medical attendants, did parents who relied on them exclusively to treat a sick or injured child fail in their legal duties? Further, if parents' failure resulted in harm to the health or life of their child, what penalties might the state impose upon them? One possibility was prosecution for manslaughter, a common law category of crimes that assigned culpability for causing the death of another person but did not require the element of intentional malice. In 1868 an English case, *Queen v. Wagstaffe*, involved the manslaughter prosecution of parents whose fourteen-month-old daughter had died from an unspecified "inflammation of the lungs." The Wagstaffes belonged to a healing sect called the Peculiar People who treated illness and injury using a religious rite involving prayer and anointing with oil. Although the little girl's parents had not sought the aid of a physician during her extended illness they had provided her with sustenance, feeding her gruel, corn flour, milk, barley water, and small amounts of brandy—apparently furnishing the latter because they believed the baby's ailment was due to teething, a reasonable assumption and parental response in the middle of the nineteenth century. The judge's charge to the jury pointed out that the Wagstaffes had remained attentive to their baby's physical needs and, further, it could not be determined whether a physician's intervention would have produced a different result given the indeterminate nature of the child's illness. The jury's decision to acquit them nevertheless sparked public controversy, resulting in Parliament revising existing laws to include clearer language defining adults' obligation to provide medical attendance to ailing children. Peters notes that medical neglect cases involving the Peculiar People continued to arise from time to time on both sides of the Atlantic. In the United States, the stronger language that had been included in the revised English law found its way into new child endangerment statutes enacted in a number of states, including the New York law under which Pierson was convicted, in the decades that followed the Wagstaffe case and its attendant public controversy.[11]

The debate surrounding faith healing and parental duties raged on in Illinois where Christian Science, like Dowie's Christian Catholic Church, was gaining a considerable following. In 1877 Illinois revised its criminal code making it unlawful for any adult having the care and custody of a child to "willfully cause or permit such child to be placed in such a situation that its life or health may be endangered." Not surprisingly, health authorities in Chicago acted with characteristic vigor, not hesitating to wield the new child endangerment law against Christian Scientist parents who eschewed regular medical treatment for their dying children. The response was particularly heated when cases involved a child's death from diphtheria and neither parents nor the healers who attended the case reported the deadly contagious disease to public health officials, an offense that garnered stiff fines under Illinois law. In 1898, for example, six-year-old Lillian Lewis died of diphtheria in the Chicago home of her Christian Scientist parents. The Cook County coroner told the *Chicago Daily Tribune* bluntly that the little girl's death represented "one of the worst cases of neglect that ever came under my observation," and, further, he had determined the child would have choked to death over an extended period of time as the pseudomembrane that was characteristic of Corynebacterium diphtheriae grew to cover the little girl's throat. He also asserted that the healthy condition of the child's organs suggested her life could have been saved by a medical operation, presumably a reference to tracheotomy or intubation. The coroner's inference here was that the child had not expired suddenly from organ failure due to the build-up of bacteriological toxins in her body, a less-expected death which might have mitigated her parents' culpability in failing to seek medical attendance in time to save the little girl's life. The following year Cook County coroners' juries censured Christian Scientist parents in two more cases, each involving a four-year-old child who died of diphtheria.[12]

But, while parents faced heightened scrutiny under the watchful eyes of regular physicians in Cook County, the state's attorney general, Edward C. Akin, hesitated to go so far as to pursue criminal charges against them. When a six-year-old boy died of typhoid fever without receiving medical treatment, for example, Akin determined that the child's Christian Scientist parents had not violated the state's criminal code because their sincerely held belief in the efficacy of their church's healers meant they had not willfully intended to harm their son. The case had occurred in rural Douglas County, more than one hundred and fifty miles south of Chicago and therefore well beyond the reach of the aggressive physicians who occupied that city's health department and the Cook County Coroner's Office. Nevertheless, Akin's cautious approach ignited a debate among members of the Illinois bar. Assistant State's Attorney John H. Lee preferred a more robust legal response to cases of medical neglect, including those involving parents who eschewed physicians for religious reasons. In a paper read before the state bar association Lee insisted that common law definitions of parents' duties allowed for criminal prosecutions when they failed to secure medical attendance for a severely ill or injured child, regardless of whether their reason for not seeking aid was secular or religious. Other attorneys argued that a more effective means to protect the physical well-being of children whose parents rejected scientific medicine lay in revising the state's medical practice statute to expressly prohibit faith healing altogether. In 1900, however, avid Christian Science critic William A. Purrington disagreed with the notion that outright bans on any religion's healing activities represented an effective remedy, warning that such heavy-handed legal approaches would only result in "cheap martyrdom" for Eddy's followers.[13]

Canadians also came face-to-face with the thorny subject of faith healing and child neglect when communities of John Alexander Dowie's followers appeared in British Columbia and Ontario. As historian James Opp explains, an ordained church elder in Victoria named Eugene Brooks faced indictment in May, 1901 following the death of a four-year-old child who had succumbed to diphtheria while under his ministrations; Claude Maltby, in fact, was the second child to die without receiving medical attendance while under the elder's care. Brooks, along with the child's father Willie Maltby, were tried on a combined total of eleven criminal charges, including several stemming from Canada's newly enacted child endangerment law. (Notably, the law did not hold the child's mother responsible because, as per the Canadian law, she was not the head of the Maltby household.) Opp notes that, during the trial, the difficulty of distinguishing between an early case of "true" diphtheria caused by the bacillus Corynebacterium diphtheriae and several other, less dangerous, childhood ailments that it resembled had muddled the prosecution's case. It remained unclear whether Claude had suffocated over a period of time due to the spread of the pseudomembrane—a process that would have been observable to those who attended the little boy—or instead had succumbed suddenly due to heart failure caused by the disease's bacterial toxins. Given these medical uncertainties, the judge determined that Maltby and Brooks could not have known the child faced imminent death and thus he found both defendants not guilty of all the charges.[14]

But the Canadian courts were not yet finished with the divine healer. Just four months later, Eugene Brooks was called to pray at the home of the Maltbys' neighbors John and Alice Rogers. Despite his ministrations the couple's three-year-old daughter Nellie succumbed to diphtheria as did their seven-month-old son Cecil a few days later. In this case prosecutors secured a manslaughter conviction for John Rogers while Eugene Brooks was found guilty of counseling Rogers to criminally neglect his children and sentenced to three months in jail. Brooks' very recent experience with Claude Maltby's illness and death from diphtheria made it difficult for the healer to contend that he could not have known Nellie's condition was dangerous. What is more, he had sent Dowie a telegram asking the divine healer to pray for the little girl, specifically mentioning she was suffering from that disease. This time the divine healer and the children's father were tried separately and, significantly, in both trials the court precluded the defense from introducing their religious beliefs as justification for their refusal to seek medical help for the children. When Brooks tried to explain his church's tenet that sickness came from sin and thus only prayer could cure it, the judge interrupted him impatiently. "Oh, you have got to use a little common sense in these things," Justice George Anthony Walkem interjected. The case attracted attention outside of British Columbia. Maintaining its dogged interest in all things associated with the controversial John Alexander Dowie, the *Chicago Daily Tribune* reported on Eugene Brooks' case, as did the *New York Times*.[15]

The convictions of Dowies' adherents in British Columbia followed closely upon the case of his follower J. Luther Pierson in Westchester County, New York. Both convictions had involved violations of recent child endangerment laws that specified a duty to secure medical attendance for severely ill children. But, if American opponents of religious-based medical neglect took heart in these outcomes, they were faced with disappointment the following year. In 1902 two cases involving Christian Scientists drew national attention, reflecting both the rapid expansion and the growing notoriety of Eddy's church in the early twentieth century. Here it is worth recalling key differences between Dowie's Christian Catholic Church and Eddy's Christian Science regarding the core tenets that informed their differing views concerning sickness and death. Significantly, Dowie's adherents did not deny the empirical reality of physical illness and injury. Rather, they believed the origin of human bodily suffering lay in sin. Thus it could only be assuaged by divine power, channeled to the sufferer by prayer and, at times, by the touch of spiritual healers who were ordained in the church. Perhaps no clearer, nor more poignant, example came in May 1902 when, as we have seen, Dowie's own daughter Esther died after suffering extensive burns sustained when she overturned a spirit lamp and caught her clothing on fire in the Zion Home located in downtown Chicago. Informing his followers of the tragic event in his periodical *Leaves of Healing*, Dowie affirmed that "there is no blame attached to anyone in the Home, or anyone else but [Esther] herself" because on a previous occasion he had expressly forbidden her to use the spirit lamp. After describing her physical injuries in suprisingly graphic detail, Dowie told mourners that his daughter had strayed from the path of virtue only once in her life, but in that one fatal moment, "the Devil struck her with that liquid fire and distilled damnation," the deadly weapon of a lamp fueled by alcohol. If the cause of Esther's bodily suffering and premature death lay in the sin of disobedience to her father, nevertheless her physical ordeal had been undeniably, and agonizingly, real.

Mary Baker Eddy, by contrast, taught that sickness and pain represented Error, illusions that stood in direct opposition to the timeless and universal Truth of God's perfection. In 1902, as legal controversies swirled around the issue of religious healing and children's medical care, a new edition of *Science and Health with Key to the Scriptures* reinforced Eddy's metaphysical doctrine: "If we concede the same reality to discord as to harmony," she wrote, "it has a lasting claim upon us... If pain is as real as the absence of pain, both must be immortal; and, if so, harmony cannot be the law of being." In other words, physical suffering cannot be openly acknowledged lest it take on a value identical to Truth. The non-corporeal essence that Eddy ascribed to children in her many editions of *Science and Health* precluded Christian Scientist parents from attending too closely to the physical symptoms of illness. Further, naming and treating specific diseases risked a malicious manifestation of parents' own fears concerning their children's state of health. The criminal cases that came to the public's attention in 1902 clearly demonstrate the dilemma of assigning legal culpability to parents who, in sincerely ascribing to Eddy's metaphysical doctrines, chose not to secure medical attendance for a dying child.[16]

In October, seven-year-old Esther Quimby died of diphtheria in Westchester County, New York. Her parents, John and Georgianna Quimby, had relied exclusively on a Christian Science healer and had also failed to report the contagious disease to local health officials. When health inspectors did arrive in the Quimby household they found that two other children were also infected with diphtheria. (Tragically, the Quimbys were no strangers to the pain of losing a child, having previously experienced the deaths of four of their seven children.) The coroners' inquest, widely covered by the press in the wake of J. Luther Pierson's criminal trial in the same county one year previously, threw tensions between physical and metaphysical constructions of childhood disease and death into sharp relief. The coroner himself testified that his examination had found "enough diphtheria to infect an entire community" in the pseudomembrane that had grown in little Esther's throat; he pointedly determined the official cause of death to be "diphtheria and Christian Science neglect." For her part, Georgiana Quimby explained to the coroner's jury that when Esther expired she had sought to "recall" her with a "life thought" but the child had "gone too far" at that point to be recovered. The Quimbys denied they had medically neglected their daughter because they had hired John Carroll Lathrop, a graduate of the Massachusetts Metaphysical College, to attend Esther's case. Questioned at the inquest, however, Lathrop refused to acknowledge that the little girl had been ill at all. When asked to identify her cause of death, the noted healer replied, "nothing." Apparently dubious of Lathrop's standing as a legitimate medical practitioner, the coroner's jury held the Quimbys over to a grand jury which subsequently indicted them, not with a misdemeanor violation under the child endangerment law, but rather under a more serious, and as yet untested, charge in the State of New York: second-degree manslaughter. Facing a criminal trial, the Quimbys found overwhelming support within the substantial Christian Scientist community that had become established in Westchester County and its environs. Both John Carroll Lathrop and his mother, Laura Lathrop, held prestigious official positions within the church in New York City and also enjoyed close personal relationships with Mary Baker Eddy. "I do not fear," John Quimby confidently told the *New York Evening Journal* at the conclusion of a community meeting held in support of their cause. "We did everything possible to save our daughter's life. Our belief in the power of God is no reason why we should be persecuted."[17]

Just one month after the Quimbys were indicted another couple, Merrill and Clara Reed of Los Angeles, California were charged with second-degree manslaughter following the death of their five-year-old daughter, also from diphtheria. Unlike the Quimbys, who had unwaveringly held to Eddy's teachings throughout their children's illnesses, the Reeds' actions had been more complicated. They called not one, but rather six different Christian Science practitioners to attend little Sarah in their home over the course of her illness. They also sought the help of a regular medical doctor, Eliza Kearney. The physician later testified in court that she had arrived at the home to find Sarah on a bed with her head thrown backward, gasping and choking for breath, a signal that indicated to the doctor the presence of the tell-tale diphtheria pseudomembrane and, even more ominously, that it had extended sufficiently to block the child's airways. Upon examining the little girl Kearney visually confirmed the pseudomembrane's presence and noted its spread upward from the child's throat through the nasal passages, causing visible bleeding through the nostrils. Given the observable signs that the child was suffering and her life was in imminent danger, Kearney warned the Reeds of the strong likelihood that Sarah was infected with diphtheria and required immediate treatment with antitoxin or she would suffocate. Kearney then swabbed the child's throat and, after leaving the Reed's home, submitted the sample to the public health department, which confirmed the presence of Corynebacterium diphtheria. With her initial diagnosis supported by laboratory analysis, Kearney telephoned the Reeds and reiterated the need to administer antitoxin to the child immediately. But the Reeds refused, explaining that they wanted their daughter to be attended solely by Christian Science practitioners. Kearney remained extremely worried about Sarah, however, and later telephoned the Reed home again to check on her condition. Much to her surprise, she was told that the child had recovered. A day later, however, the Reeds asked Kearney to sign Sarah's death certificate, which she refused to do, insisting that she had not been the attending physician in the case.[18]

At the Reeds' subsequent criminal trial Los Angeles City Attorney Harley Shaw explained to the jury that under California law "a man may be guilty of manslaughter under some circumstances by mere carelessness." He asserted that, given Sarah's observable physical suffering, the doctor's clear and direct warning to the Reeds, and the laboratory's confirmation of Kearney's initial diagnosis of diphtheria, these parents not only had been careless, they had been nothing short of reckless in refusing antitoxin for their daughter. While Shaw did not deny the sincerity of the Reeds' religious beliefs, nor their "undoubted desire for their daughter's recovery," nevertheless their choice to treat her dire condition using only metaphysical means "did not take the place of the [medical] assistance she may have had for the asking." In the State of California, Shaw concluded, the Reeds' failure to procure antitoxin for their clearly distressed child met the necessary conditions for a manslaughter conviction. A prominent California attorney named Christopher C. Wright defended the Reeds. He employed a bold strategy that countered the state's forensic case with what amounted to an exegesis of Mary Baker Eddy's treatise *Science and Health*. Called to the witness stand, one of Sarah's attendants insisted that the appearance of choking indicated, not the presence of the pseudomembrane in the child's body, but rather the "inharmoniousness" caused by the "crude state" of her parents' understanding. "Death," she explained to the jury, "is the manifestation of the carnal mind." Another healer who had seen Sarah within twenty minutes of her death denied she had been ill at all, insisting the child was "getting along nicely and seemed bright enough." A third practitioner explained that diphtheria antitoxin itself served as a medium for the spread Error; she claimed she had once contracted diphtheria when antitoxin was administered to another person in her presence. After the testimony from Sarah's attendants, Wright called a panoply of additional witnesses—over the vociferous objections of the prosecutor. Although completely unrelated to Sarah's case, their testimony described their own successful healings under Christian Science. By introducing extensive anecdotes in support of the effectiveness of Eddy's metaphysical healing paradigm, Wright deflected the jury's focus away from the damning physical evidence provided by the actual body of Sarah Reed. One journalist commented that the court heard so many miraculous healing accounts that the victim herself seemed to drop out of the case entirely. Wright framed Christian Science and diphtheria antitoxin as equivalent therapeutic options and the Reeds' responses as reasonable parental choices under the circumstances of their daughter's illness. The jury voted for acquittal. Remarking on the trial's outcome, the *Los Angeles Times* noted with incredulity that the state had presented a case based on material facts, only to be bested by the defense's denial that material facts even exist.[19]

The dismissal of manslaughter charges against the Reeds undoubtedly boosted the Quimbys' fortunes three thousand miles away in Westchester County, New York. Before their trial commenced, the couple had filed a demurrer arguing that a jury made up of lay people could not possibly determine whether the Christian Scientist practitioner John Lathrop's metaphysical ministrations were any less effective (and therefore the Quimbys' choice to employ him any less reasonable) than the interventions of a mainstream medical doctor. Perhaps of equal significance to the Quimby's argument were two laboratory debacles that had recently unfolded beginning in November 1901. Tragically, thirteen children died of tetanus after receiving contaminated diphtheria antitoxin in St. Louis, Missouri and, several months later, nine more children died under the same circumstances in Camden, New Jersey. (In 1902 Congress used its constitutional powers to regulate interstate commerce in passing the Biologics Control Act, which allowed the federal government increased scrutiny and control over the production of antitoxin and vaccines. Supporters argued the measure was necessary because most cities purchased antitoxin that was manufactured out of state. The federal Food and Drug Administration was created four years later.) The horrific national scandal served to reinforce the notion that, despite notable progress in the science of bacteriology and the perhaps-outsized hopes it had inspired, medical science still had far to go in alleviating the uncertainties that surrounded childhood disease and death at the turn of the twentieth century. In 1905, three years after the Quimbys filed their demurrer, a New York County judge finally agreed and dismissed their case. For Judge William P. Platt, the "standard for determining what was proper and necessary medical care was too variable for the allegation [of second-degree manslaughter] to be used as the description of a definite act." For Judge Platt, the significant fact was that the cause of Esther Quimby's death had been diphtheria, not the parental choices that John and Georgiana Quimby had made in response to their daughter's illness. American courts remained wary of subjecting parents who had lost their children to the additional hardship of serious criminal penalties; manslaughter convictions were also overturned on appeal in Indiana (1904), Maine (1905), and New Jersey (1909).[20]

By contrast, in 1907 a New York court sentenced Christian Scientist Clarence W. Byrne to thirty days in jail under the same child endangerment statute that had been used to successfully prosecute J. Luther Pierson six years previously. Byrne, a department store sales clerk, had been tried following the death of his six-year-old daughter Violet from bronchial pneumonia. Unlike Pierson, who told the court he was aware his child had been seriously ill, Byrne never acknowledged his daughter to be sick at all. He had engaged a Christian Science practitioner who employed the technique of "absent treatment," mentally arguing against the Error of Violet's sickness in order to replace it with the Truth that she was in perfect health. This form of medical attendance had been exercised from a distance, without the healer ever observing, or even being in the presence of, the ailing child. On the witness stand Byrne objected to the court's continual use of the word "died" in reference to Violet, insisting that "Christian Scientists know no death... there is only dissolution." A three-judge panel of the Court of Special Sessions found Byrne guilty of violating the state's child neglect law, ruling that his choice to employ absent treatment exclusively despite signs indicating that Violet was seriously ill had placed his daughter in danger. Significantly, the judges noted that they found it "extremely vexatious" to contemplate ever allowing a parent to plead a religious disbelief that his child possessed a physical body as an excuse for withholding food, clothing, or shelter—parental duties already well established under common law. For this court Byrne's denial of mainstream medical care to his gravely ill daughter had been no different than denying her any of the other "necessaries" required to sustain her life. Editorializing on the Byrne case, the *New York Times* pointedly observed that the "absent treatment" upon which this father had relied consisted of nothing more than an "assertion that nothing can be the matter with the patient and denial that there is anything for the matter" of dealing with the patient's physically compromised state.[21]

By 1910, then, a discernible pattern had emerged. While specific statutory language differed among individual states, American courts were generally disinclined to allow parents to be convicted on manslaughter charges when they eschewed physicians' services for their dying children as a matter of religious faith. While scientific medicine showed much promise in mitigating the deadly diseases of childhood, it could not establish a bright line of certainty that a child's death had been caused by a parent's actions (or inaction) rather than by the fact that the child had had the misfortune to contract a fatal disease. Courts were more likely, however, to uphold convictions under states' newly enacted child abuse and neglect laws that expressly defined a parental duty to secure medical attendance when circumstances warranted that they do so. Enacted in the last quarter of the nineteenth century, these statutes reflected broader changes in Americans' sensibilities regarding the significance of children's physical growth and development and their need for specialized attention and care. Further, several courts expressly rejected the notion that a belief in religious or metaphysical forms of healing, even if sincerely held by parents, could serve as a defense to the charge of endangering a child when a young victim had suffered observable, life-threatening physical symptoms. The trend was reinforced in 1911, for example, when the Oklahoma Supreme Court upheld a father's conviction under that state's medical neglect law. At trial Lawrence Owens acknowledged that he knew his daughter to be seriously ill with typhoid fever but nevertheless had eschewed medical attendance for her due to his religious faith. "Under the law in this state, there is probably no way of reaching an adult who refuses to accept medical aid for himself on his own responsibility," the justices surmised. "But under the statute… persons will not be permitted to allow innocent children, [who are] dependent upon them, to suffer for the lack of necessary food, clothing, shelter, or medical attendance." The Oklahoma statute, like those in many other states, specifically included medical attendance among the "necessaries" that adults owed to children. In the meantime, public attention to children's physical welfare continued to gain momentum in the early twentieth century, as evidenced by the formation of the American Association for the Study and Prevention of Infant Mortality in 1908 and the Child Health Organization in 1917.[22]

In response, advocates of religious healing, most particularly Christian Scientists, organized to form a substantial movement of their own to resist the trend linking children's medical care to the growth of states' police powers. "Who is to decide this question?" inquired a 1906 publication by the Christian Science church. "Shall it be decided beforehand by the majority of a group of gentlemen under the gilded dome of a State-house? Or shall the choice be left with the child's parents, who are its natural guardians, who are at the bedside and to whom the little one's life means more than it does to all other persons?" As historian Rennie E. Schoepflin explained, the church's Committees on Publication, established by Mary Baker Eddy in 1898, became a powerful lobbying wing of the institutional church with members assigned to monitor and influence legislatures in every state as well as in several major cities. The Committee's initial goals were to ensure special exemptions for religious healing within state medical licensing laws and to push back against states' expanding use of their police powers to enforce public health measures such as compulsory vaccination against smallpox. In such efforts Christian Scientists were joined by secular medical dissenters including those who in 1910 formed the National League for Medical Freedom. The League dedicated itself to challenging state laws it characterized as "unjust, oppressive, paternal and un-American," and to resisting the regular medical establishment's efforts to "make the Government an immense anthropomorphic and allopathic physician." Even Mark Twain, a caustic critic of Mary Baker Eddy who had himself experienced the loss of a beloved child (a tragedy some attributed to his wife's interest in Christian Science), chastised those who would dare to presume upon a father's prerogatives. "It is a burning shame," Twain wrote mockingly in 1907, "that the law does not require him to come to *me* to ask what kind of healer I will allow him to call." Twain's humor notwithstanding, reframing the issue as one of individual autonomy and religious liberty–rather than as the child's right to receive medical attendance in accordance with the "science of the age"—proved to be a powerful, and persistent, counterargument, one that lingered in the background of American life for the remainder of the twentieth century.[23]

## NOTES

1. *New York v. J. Luther Pierson* 176 N.Y. 201; 68 N.E. 243; 1903; "Topics of the Times," *New York Times* (May 23, 1901): 8; "A Faith Curist Sentenced," *Chicago Daily Tribune* (May 24, 1901): 12; "Dowie, Simpson,

and Their Genus," *Christian Advocate* (May 30, 1901): 846. Contrary
to his previous proclamations asserting parents' religious rights, Dowie
distanced himself from Pierson's predicament, telling readers of *Leaves of
Healing* that he had "nothing to do with" the case and, in fact, "Mr. Pierson chose to become a member of our church two weeks before his child
died." At his trial, however, Pierson told the court he had been a church
member for five years. See: "An Erroneous Decision of the Supreme Court
of New York," *Leaves of Healing*, Volume XIV, Number 4 (November 14,
1903): 112. Pierson's lawyer tried to collect $1000 in legal fees he claimed
to be owed by the Dowie's church. "Dowie's Baggage Attached," *New
York Times* (October 25, 1903): 8.

2. *New York v. J. Luther Pierson* 80 A.D. 415; N.Y.S. 214 1903; "Willard
Bartlett," http://www.nycourts.gov.

3. *New York v. J. Luther Pierson*; "William W. Goodrich," http://www.
nycourts.gov. On pertussis, see Samuel H. Preston and Michael R. Haines,
*Fatal Years: Child Mortality in Late Nineteenth-Century America* (Princeton: Princeton University Press, 1991), 18–19; "Treatment of Whooping Cough," *Journal of the American Medical Association*, Volume XXXIV
(April 28, 1900): 1059.

4. *New York v. J. Luther Pierson* 176 N.Y. 201; 68 N.E. 243; 1903. The case
Judge Haight cited is *Edward Cowley, Plaintiff in Error, v. The People of the
State of New York, Defendant in Error* 83 N.Y. 464; 1881; "Faith Cure a
Crime," *Chicago Daily Tribune* (October 14, 1903): 1; "Murder Declared
Unlawful," *New York Times* (October 15, 1903): 8. For his part, Pierson
saw no reason to modify his own convictions eschewing scientific medicine.
The *New York Times* subsequently reported a second child's death as well as
that of an unrelated adult woman in Pierson's household. "Criminal Faith
Healing," *New York Times* (October 14, 1903): 1.

5. James D. Schmidt, *Industrial Violence and the Legal Origins of Child
Labor* (New York: Cambridge University Press, 2010); Stephen Robertson, *Crimes Against Children: Sexual Violence and Legal Culture in New
York City, 1880–1960* (Chapel Hill: University of North Carolina Press,
2005).

6. William Blackstone, *Commentaries on the Laws of England*, Volume I,
446–454. Reprinted in Robert H. Mnookin and D. Kelly Weisberg, editors, *Child, Family, and State* (Aspen Publishers, 2000), 255–259; Mark E.
Brandon, *States of Union: Families and Change in the American Constitutional Order* (Lawrence: University of Kansas Press, 2013), 44; Ruth Wallis
Herndon, "'Proper' Magistrates and Masters: Binding Out Poor Children
in Southern New England, 1720–1820." In Ruth Wallis Herndon and John
E. Murray, editors, *Children Bound to Labor: The Pauper Apprentice System
in Early America* (Ithaca: Cornell University Press, 2009), 39–51.

7. Michael Grossberg, *Governing the Hearth: Law and the Family in Nineteenth-Century America* (University of North Carolina Press, 1985), 237–286; Mary Ann Mason, *From Father's Property to Children's Rights: The History of Child Custody in the United States* (New York: Columbia University Press, 1994), 49–84; James Schouler, *A Treatise on the Law of Domestic Relations* (Boston: Little, Brown and Company, 1870), 548; David S. Tanenhaus, "Between Dependency and Liberty: The Conundrum of Children's Rights in the Gilded Age," *Law and History Review*, Volume 23 Number 2 (Summer 2005): 351–385; Nancy Hathaway Steenburg, *Children and the Criminal Law in Connecticut, 1635–1855: Changing Perceptions of Childhood* (New York: Routledge, 2005), 132.

8. *Reynolds v. United States* 98 U.S. 145, 1878.

9. *Dent v. State of West Virginia* 9 S. Ct. 231, 1889. On eclectic medicine see William G. Rothstein, "The Botanical Movements and Orthodox Medicine." In Norman Gevitz, editor, *Other Healers: Unorthodox Medicine in America* (Baltimore: Johns Hopkins University Press, 1988), 29–51.

10. *State v. Buswell* 40 Neb. 158 1894; *State v. Mylod* 20 R. I. 632 1898; "An Important Decision," *Christian Science Journal* Volume 16 (September 1898): 405–416; "Construction of a Statute. Practice of Medicine. Christian Science. State v. Mylod 40 Atl. Rep. (R.I.) 753," *The Yale Law Journal*, Volume 8, Number 1 (October 1898): 57; *Commonwealth v. Thomson* 6 Mass 134 1809; William A. Purrington, *A Review of Recent Legal Decisions Affecting Physicians, Dentists, Druggists and the Public Health* (New York: E.B. Treat and Company, 1899), 105; "X-Practice Declared Legal," *Quincy Daily Whig* (October 9, 1904): 2.

11. Shawn Francis Peters, *When Prayer Fails: Faith Healing, Children, and the Law* (New York: Oxford University Press, 47–66.

12. Merritt Starr and Russell H. Curtis, editors, *Annotated Statutes of the State of Illinois*, Volume I (Chicago: Callahan and Company, 1885), 770; "Follows Up Faith Cure Cases," *Chicago Daily Tribune* (June 2, 1899): 10; "May Indict Scientist Parents" *Chicago Daily Tribune* (June 3, 1899): 16; "To Act in Diphtheria Case," *Chicago Daily Tribune* (June 4, 1899): 3; "Christian Science Fails to Save Life of Lillian Lewis," *Chicago Daily Tribune* (October 23, 1899): 12.

13. "Children the Victims," *Chicago Daily Tribune* (September 10, 1899): 32; "Say Repeal if Akin is Right," *Chicago Daily Tribune* (September 10, 1899): 8; "Combine Crowds Out Individual," *Chicago Daily Tribune* (July 13, 1901): 7; William A. Purrington, *Christian Science* (New York: E.B. Treat and Company, 1900), 34.

14. James Opp, *The Lord for the Body: Religion, Medicine, and Protestant Faith Healing in Canada, 1880–1930* (Montreal: McGill-Queen's University Press, 2005), 91–110.

15. Opp, *The Lord for the Body*, 110–120; "E Brooks, A Dowie Zionist, Sentenced," *New York Times* (November 26, 1901): 2; "Sentence Dowieite to Prison," *Chicago Daily Tribune* (November 26, 1901): 2.

16. "Story of the Fatal Injury and Triumphant Departure," *Leaves of Healing*, Volume XI, Number 4 (May 17, 1902): 107–115; Mary Baker G. Eddy, *Science and Health with Key to the Scriptures* (Boston: Joseph A. Armstrong, 1902), 186.

17. "Child Died Without Medical Attendance," *New York Times* (October 22, 1902): 16; "Scientists' Defy Coroner," *The World* (October 22, 1902): 5; "Inquest in Quimby Case," *New York Daily Tribune* (October 22, 1902): 6; "Faith Healers are Locked Up," *The World* (October 23, 1902): 1; "How Prayer Failed to Cure Diphtheria," *New York Times* (October 23, 1902): "Christian Scientists Held for Manslaughter," *New York Times* (October 24, 1902): 1; "Healer and Father Held," *New York Daily Tribune* (October 24, 1902): 3; "Christian Scientists Must Stand Trial," *New York* Times (October 31, 1902); "Healers Call Mass Meeting for Quimbys," *New York Evening Journal* (October 25, 1902). John Carroll Lathrop's name appears in a list of graduates of the Massachusetts Metaphysical College. Records of the Massachusetts Metaphysical College, Box #156, Folder "1886 Curriculum." The Mary Baker Eddy Library, Boston, MA.

18. "Christian Scientists in Meshes of Law," *Los Angeles Times* (November 26, 1902); "Child Died Under Christian Science," *Los Angeles Times* (November 27, 1902).

19. "Christian Scientists Won a Verdict," *Los Angeles Times* (November 30, 1902); *Criminal Law and Procedure of California* (Los Angeles: Charles W. Balm Co., 1902), 180–182; *The Los Angeles Case; The People Versus Merrill Reed et al.* (Boston: The Christian Science Publishing Society, 1904); "Christopher C. Wright." Wellington C. Wolfe, editor, *Men of California* (San Francisco: The Pacific Art Company, 1901), 107.

20. *People v. Quimby* 113 App. Div. 793 (N.Y. App. Div. 1906). In St. Louis the coroner's office held an extensive inquiry and, subsequently, a special Court of Inquiry held the city bacteriologist, Armand Revold, as well as a janitor named Henry Taylor responsible and dismissed both men. The city also ceased producing serum in its own public health laboratory: "Did Horse with Tetanus Furnish Antitoxin Serum?" *St. Louis Republic* (November 3, 1901): 1; "Dr. Ravold Declares Bacteriologists Have Erred," *St. Louis Republic* (November 19, 1901): 1; "Virus and Antitoxin of the Health Board," *New York Times* (November 24, 1901): 5; "Taylor Admits Having Issued Toxic Serum," *St. Louis Republic* (December 27, 1901): 1; "The Antitoxin Scandal in St. Louis," *New York Times* (February 14, 1902): 8; Ross E. DeHovitz, "The 1901 St. Louis Incident: The First Modern Medical Disaster," *Pediatrics*, Volume 133, Number 6 (June 2014): 964–965.

21. "Jury Would Make Eddyism a Felony," *New York Times* (May 18, 1907): 1; "Jail Sentence for Eddyite," *New York Times* (August 3, 1907): 14; "Mr. Byrne Counts for Little," *New York Times* (August 5, 1907): 6; "Christian Science Wins," *New York Times* (February 24, 1909): 5; Robert L. Trescher and Thomas N. O'Neill, Jr., "Medical Care for Dependent Children: Manslaughter Liability of the Christian Scientist," *University of Pennsylvania Law Review*, Volume 109 (1960): 203–217. Fascinating context for the Maine case involving divine healer Frank Weston Sandford is provided in Shirley Nelson, *Fair, Clear, and Terrible: The Story of Shiloh* (Eugene, OR: Wipf and Stock 2009).

22. *Owens v. State* 6 Okla. Crim. 110, 116 Pac. 345 (1911). Not all states followed the general pattern. In 1902, for example, the Georgia Supreme Court struck down a father's conviction for violating that state's child neglect law, which stipulated only a duty to provide "sustenance," arguing that the legislature had not intended medicine to be included within the category of "sustenance." *Bennett v. Ware*, 4 Ga A. 293, 61 S.E. 546.

23. Claire Hoertz Badaracco, *Prescribing Faith: Medicine, Media, and Religion in American Culture* (Baylor University Press, 2007), 61; *Christian Science and Legislation* (The Christian Science Publishing Company, 1906), 42; Rennie B. Schoepflin, *Christian Science on Trial: Religious Healing in America* (Baltimore: Johns Hopkins University Press, 2003), 161–167; *The Facts About "Colliers'" Attack on the National League for Medical Freedom* (National League for Medical Freedom, no date), no page number; Mark Twain, *Christian Science* (Elibron Classics, 2006), 48.

# CHAPTER 8

# The Science of the Age

Shall a parent, who belongs to that exemplary band of Christians who have no faith in the efficacy of medicine as a curative agency, be convicted of manslaughter, because he fails to call a physician to attend a sick child that subsequently dies? Until the practice of medicine becomes an exact science so that it can be established beyond the peradventure of a doubt that death would not have ensued if a physician had been in attendance, I think the answer to all these questions must be an unqualified, "No."

In 1920 the Supreme Court of Florida overturned the manslaughter conviction of James Bradley in the death of his daughter Bertha. The sixteen-year-old had sustained severe burns after falling into a fire while experiencing an epileptic seizure. Bradley, an adherent of divine healing, had refused to seek medical attendance for the girl during a period extending over two months. "All the doctor I want is Jesus," Bradley had affirmed to witnesses, a firm spiritual commitment that included rejecting the help of local Red Cross nurses who offered to dress the child's wounds and provide palliative care during her long ordeal. Ultimately, Bertha was removed to the Florida Hospital for the Insane by order of the local justice of the peace. The justice's help had been solicited by Bradley's brother-in-law who had witnessed the girl's prolonged suffering and later testified that what he had seen "made me so mad that I could hardly stand it." Bertha died

© The Author(s) 2019
L. Curry, *Religion, Law, and the Medical Neglect
of Children in the United States, 1870–2000*,
Palgrave Studies in the History of Childhood,
https://doi.org/10.1007/978-3-030-24689-1_8

while in the custody of the hospital. Physicians who attended her there told the criminal court that, in their opinion, had she received prompt medical attention at the time of the accident Bertha would have recovered. The Florida Supreme Court, however, didn't share the physicians' faith in the efficacy of their professional efforts. Because regular medicine was not, as yet, an "exact science," the court reasoned, it remained the case that "the attentions of a physician may or may not have prevented the burning from causing the death of the child." Bertha died as a result of the injuries she had sustained, not from the actions taken by her father; James Bradley's conviction under Florida's manslaughter statute therefore could not be upheld.[1]

Justice Thomas F. West wrote a lone dissent in the case, basing his reasoning on language that defined manslaughter in the State of Florida as "the killing of a human being by the act, procurement or culpable negligence of another." By Justice West's reckoning, Bradley's steadfast refusal to seek medical attention for his daughter despite his awareness of her dire condition did, in fact, fall within the meaning of the statute. Citing Schouler's 1870 work, *A Treatise on the Law of Domestic Relations* and Justice Albert Haight's opinion in *People v. Pierson*, written nearly twenty years previously, West maintained it was a "well settled" matter that "it is the legal duty of a father, who is able to do so, to furnish necessary medical attention for his child." For this justice, it was not necessary for the court to wait for a future date when regular medicine became an "exact science." Rather, in the State of Florida, in the year 1920, it was a well-established parental duty to provide medical attendance to a sick or injured child and thus Bradley's refusal to do so constituted "culpable negligence" that had resulted in Bertha's death. "The [trial jury's] verdict is amply supported by the evidence," West noted, and thus this father's manslaughter conviction should be affirmed.[2]

The divine healer John Alexander Dowie died in 1907, followed by Christian Science founder Mary Baker Eddy three years later. Yet, as the conflicting perspectives articulated by the justices of the Florida Supreme Court in 1920 illustrate, the discursive framing of the debate concerning children's physical well-being, and the duties imposed upon the adults who are responsible for them, endured beyond these influential religious leaders' own lifetimes. Both Dowie and Eddy had drawn considerable followings through their message that medical science, fallible and subject to change, could not be trusted. True and lasting healing came only through spiritual means, which were universal and eternal. The claim for spiritual over temporal healing, however, became increasingly hard to sustain as the early promise of bacteriology in the late nineteenth century finally came to fruition in the first half of the twentieth. In 1913 the German physiologist Emil Behring derived a toxin-antitoxin formulation that, unlike the emergency use of antitoxin once diphtheria had been contracted, provided long-lasting immunity from this deadly childhood disease. In the same year the Austrian physician Bela Schick derived a skin test to determine the presence of diphtheria antibodies, making it possible to measure the efficacy of the new vaccine. In the United States the practical application of bacteriological research led to the licensing and production of vaccines offering immunity from long-dreaded childhood scourges such as tetanus and pertussis. Within ten years new understandings of childhood diseases emanating from European laboratories had worked their way into standard medical texts used to train regular physicians. Just as significantly, public perceptions of the value of scientific medicine for children's health were changing as well. Decades of vigorous child welfare campaigns had disseminated the germ theory among a popular audience, raising awareness of the potential life-saving benefits to young children when the adults who cared for them observed hygienic measures such as frequent handwashing, screening windows to protect against germ-carrying flies, and feeding babies pasteurized milk in sterilized bottles. Pediatricians' close association with turn-of-the-century child welfare campaigns had brought thousands of parents in contact with this emerging cadre of medical professionals The new medical specialty entered a growth phase as pediatricians expanded their domain to include supervising children's normal growth and development in addition to managing the deadly diseases of childhood. In 1933 the American Board of Pediatrics was established as a national certifying body that examined physicians' competency as specialists in children's health care. As scientific medicine penetrated an ever-expanding number of households Mary Baker Eddy's metaphysical paradigm of health and illness, with its origins in early nineteenth-century ether theories, began to appear outmoded and indeed eccentric by comparison. For the first time since its founding, between 1930 and 1940 her church's rate of growth began to slow down.[3]

Tensions between spiritual and scientific healing had already led to several concessions from religious leaders. Both Dowie and Eddy had authorized vaccination and urged cooperation with public health authorities when smallpox broke out in communities of the faithful. Shortly before her death Eddy modified her antipathy toward *materia medica* to allow morphine for pain control. After 1910, as the twentieth century progressed without their church's leader, Christian Scientists continued to make compromises, and by the mid-twentieth century dwindling numbers took the hard line that church members called "radical reliance," eschewing the use of all scientific medicine for themselves as well as for their children. Official church publications, however, continued to construe diseases as Error, false perceptions rather than biological facts. The healing methods employed by the church's certified practitioners, including silent argumentation and absent treatment, remained unchanged since Eddy opened the Massachusetts Metaphysical College in 1881. Although the church insisted that its members were always free to follow their own consciences in making medical decisions, critics charged that community pressure to rely on Christian Science healing alone remained influential in shaping parents' responses when their children fell ill.[4]

As spiritual healing became increasingly difficult to justify on the grounds of its equivalence to scientific medicine, proponents relied more heavily on the argument that parental decisions regarding their children's well-being constituted matters of religious freedom. In the late nineteenth century Christian Scientists had been instrumental in the enactment of legislation excepting spiritual healers from the more rigorous education and training requirements that states had begun to require for medical licensure. The church now sought to build upon these early legislative successes by pursuing a variety of additional exemptions for its own practices. Several states excused the children of Christian Scientists from undergoing school medical examinations and from attending health and hygiene classes, and some released school employees from mandatory tuberculosis testing. As the church's numbers declined, the Committees on Publication adopted a strategy that minimized Christian Scientists' doctrinal differences with mainstream Protestants, linking Eddy's metaphysical healing system to scriptural references and stressing its direct continuity with the practices of early Christians. As historian Shawn Francis Peters observed, church leaders insisted that Christian Scientists were "dutiful citizens rather than peculiar cultists" and asserted that all Americans shared an interest in the protection of religious liberty. Objections to special statutory exemptions for their practices, they argued, amounted to anti-religious bigotry.[5]

Signals from the U.S. Supreme Court suggested the wisdom of taking such an approach. While the First Amendment to the Constitution protected the "free exercise" of religion, in 1878 Chief Justice Morrison R. Waite's opinion in *Reynolds v. U.S.* had drawn a clear distinction between religious beliefs and religious practices, determining that while the First Amendment protected the former, state and federal governments enjoyed wider leeway in regulating the latter. Fifty years later, however, the court appeared to be edging toward a more nuanced perspective. In 1925 a unanimous court in *Pierce v. Society of Sisters* ruled that an Oregon law requiring public schooling violated parents' liberty to send their children to religious institutions. In 1944 the U.S. Supreme Court again reconsidered constitutional protections for religious practices. In *Prince v. Massachusetts*, an ordained minister of the Jehovah's Witnesses had been convicted of violating that state's law prohibiting children from engaging in street trades. Sarah Prince allowed her own two sons, as well as her nine-year-old ward, to accompany her in selling church publications on the streets of Brockton. In a five-to-four decision, the Court narrowly rejected Prince's claim that, because Jehovah's Witnesses regarded selling the magazines as integral to the evangelization work required by their faith, that activity must enjoy constitutional protection under the free exercise clause. Writing for the majority, Justice Wiley B. Rutledge was careful to acknowledge the essential importance of parents' liberty of conscience in raising their offspring. But he also recognized that states had an essential role to play in protecting children's health and safety. "A democratic society rests, for its continuance," Justice Rutledge wrote, "upon the healthy, well-rounded growth of young people into full maturity as citizens, with all that implies." He addressed Sarah Prince's claim by insisting that "parents may be free to become martyrs themselves. But it does not follow they are free, in identical circumstances, to make martyrs of their children before they have reached the age of full and legal discretion when they can make that choice for themselves." American courts subsequently built upon the *Prince* precedent to intervene in cases involving Jehovah's Witness parents who objected to blood transfusions as a tenet of their faith, overriding parents' wishes and permitting hospitals to use the procedure to save the lives of seriously injured children. Nevertheless, while Chief Justice Rutledge had strongly affirmed the state's role in safeguarding children's well-being, the court was badly split on the decision, indicating their wariness about allowing states to intrude too far on parental prerogatives. Writing in dissent, Justice Frank Murphy argued that children selling magazines in the early evening hours while accompanied by a parent hardly posed the kind of health and safety risk that the Massachusetts' law—aimed at unsupervised newsboys, boot blacks, and street performers—was intended to safeguard against. Taking note of the unfortunate fact that Jehovah's Witnesses already had been subjected to vigilante harassment and violence, Justice Murphy warned that allowing states too much latitude without clearly defined benefits to children's welfare risked making child labor laws into an instrument of oppression to be wielded against members of an unpopular religion.[6]

The trajectory of expanding protections for religious practices continued after World War II. In 1963 the Supreme Court ruled that South Carolina had placed a "significant burden" on the free exercise of religion by denying unemployment benefits to Adell Sherbert, a Seventh-Day Adventist who had lost her job for refusing to work on Saturday, her church's sabbath. "To condition the availability of benefits upon [Sherbert's] willingness to violate a cardinal principle of her religious faith effectively penalizes the free exercise of her constitutional liberties," Justice William Brennan wrote in *Sherbert v. Verner*. Nine years later, the court ruled that a Wisconsin law compelling school attendance after the eighth grade also infringed upon the free exercise of religion. In *Wisconsin v. Yoder* the court argued that the Old Order Amish community's objections to the state's requirement were firmly grounded in the tenets of their faith, which required parents to shield their children from worldly influence. Wisconsin had argued that it was acting in the state's long-established role as *parens patriae* in extending mandatory education to the high school level. But Chief Justice Warren Burger rejected that claim, asserting that the state had not clearly demonstrated that Amish children's welfare would be compromised if their formal education ended at the eighth grade. The Amish community was centered around agriculture, Burger noted, and for generations parents had trained older children to take up their adult roles on the farm. Interestingly, the Chief Justice expressly denied that the agricultural labor Amish children performed could be "in any way deleterious to their health."[7]

Courts were firmer in supporting state action when the benefit to the public's health and safety was easier to discern. By mid-century, as the historical terror of smallpox contagion faded from the public's consciousness, a mysterious new disease took its place. Polio had been virtually unknown in the United States prior to the late 1800s. For decades the viral disease puzzled and frustrated researchers seeking to pinpoint how, exactly, it was transmitted between individuals. Contrary to a prevailing wisdom that assumed higher socioeconomic class standing protected households from "filth" diseases such as dysentery and typhoid, polio struck wealthy and middle-class families as often as poor ones, a seeming anomaly that had led epidemiologists down numerous dead-ends. While in the vast majority of cases the infected person experienced flu-like symptoms but went on to fully recover, in about one percent of cases the patient suffered permanent paralysis. In 1952 alone over twenty-one thousand people in the United States were left paralyzed by the disease. Localities throughout the nation closed down public parks and swimming pools and frightened parents kept their children indoors. Historian James Colgrove noted that, given the context of fear and uncertainty that surrounded polio at mid-century, the launch of the Salk vaccine in 1954 brought about an unprecedented public regard for medicine as "a valuable national asset and force for the betterment of humanity." That good opinion was shared by the courts, which enthusiastically backed the use of the new vaccine to prevent polio's spread. In 1957, for example, a superior court in Chicago granted a father's request that his seven-year-old daughter be vaccinated over the objections of the child's mother, who was a Christian Scientist. Two years later the New Jersey Superior Court allowed local boards to require that children receive polio immunizations in order to attend public schools.[8]

In contrast, the legal system was more likely to defer to parental rights when containing a dangerous disease was not an issue. In 1956, Edward and Anna Cornelius of Swarthmore, Pennsylvania faced charges of involuntary manslaughter in the death of their son. When seven-year-old David became seriously ill his parents took him to a local hospital where he was diagnosed with juvenile diabetes. Upon his discharge, a physician warned that the boy required daily insulin injections in order to survive. The couple placed their son in a Christian Science nursing home in Philadelphia where, without insulin therapy, he fell into a coma and died. Although a grand jury indicted the Corneliuses on charges of involuntary manslaughter, the district attorney had several reservations about the wisdom of taking their case to trial. The nursing home was licensed by the state of Pennsylvania, suggesting the state was fully aware that the tenets of Christian Science precluded the administration of insulin to diabetic patients and therefore the Corneliuses had broken no laws in choosing the facility. Further, Pennsylvania had enacted a number of religious exemptions pertaining to health and medical care. Couples citing religious objections, for example, were excused from taking a blood test that was required to obtain a marriage license. Finally, David's untreated juvenile diabetes was in no way contagious and therefore it had posed no discernible threat to the health of other children. Wagering that such circumstances made a conviction in the case unlikely, the district attorney petitioned the court to drop the charges, a motion that Pennsylvania law required in order to stop a case from going forward. In granting the petition Judge Theodore L. Reimel presented a ringing endorsement of parents' religious liberty, declaring broadly that "if the failure to provide medical care is the result of religious tenet or a sincere belief in the inefficacy of medical treatment there may be no criminal responsibility under the law."[9]

But addressing the issue of spiritual healing solely as the free exercise of religion shifted the focus of attention away from the bodies of sick and injured children and blunted discussions about how their physical care could be most effectively—or even humanely—addressed. The problem resurfaced dramatically in 1967 when a five-year-old girl died in Cape Cod, Massachusetts of bacterial pneumonia that had developed from strep throat. Over a period of three weeks Dorothy Sheridan had treated her daughter in accordance with Christian Science practice by silently arguing against the claim of illness and reading aloud to the child from *Science and Health with Key to the Scriptures*. She had also employed the services of a Christian Science practitioner and, when Lisa's condition did not appear to improve, she had contacted a second healer who treated the child using absent treatment. Lisa died very early one morning but Sheridan waited over five hours before calling a local funeral home director. Upon learning that a death certificate had not been signed by a physician, the director followed legal protocol and called the police as well as the medical examiner to the home. Obtaining information for the death certificate, the medical examiner found Sheridan's answers to his questions about Lisa's care during her illness puzzling; he was also suspicious about the length of time that had passed between her death and the call to the funeral home. He decided that an autopsy was required, which was carried out over Dorothy Sheridan's objections. The medical examiner determined that Lisa's cause of death had been suffocation caused by empyema, or an accumulation of pus in the pleural cavity, which in fact had become so massive it had displaced her diaphragm and collapsed her right lung. Dorothy Sheridan was indicted on a charge of manslaughter.[10]

After several decades of relative quiet, Sheridan's well-publicized case renewed public controversy over Christian Scientists' rejection of scientific medicine when their children fell ill. Alarmed by the potential damage, the church supplied Sheridan's legal counsel, and ultimately mounted a defense of Christian Science itself. At the trial the medical examiner stated that Lisa's life was likely to have been spared had she been given antibiotics, used to treat streptococcal infections since the 1940s. The medical examiner also believed that, even at a late stage in the child's long illness, a surgical operation to drain the affected areas was likely to have succeeded in saving her life.

The defense countered with testimony from a pediatrician who explained the difficulty of determining whether an illness was caused by streptococcus or staphylococcus bacteria, which were often present simultaneously in major infections, the latter being much less responsive to treatment with antibiotics. The testimony suggested that, because regular medicine remained an inexact science, the jury could not determine with certainty that a physician's attention would have saved Lisa's life. The pediatrician, however, also described several interventions that he himself would have attempted had Lisa Sheridan been his patient, thereby undercutting the defense's purpose. The medical experts were followed by several prominent Christian Scientists who held prestigious positions throughout the United States, a strategy intended to establish that Dorothy Sheridan was not an eccentric character but rather a member of established and respected religion. Finally, the defense noted that Massachusetts law required parents to furnish "proper physical care" but did not specify that such care must be expressly "medical" in nature.[11]

In instructing the jury, however, Judge Eugene A. Hudson said that the statutory language referring to "proper physical care" meant the care of the child's body, and therefore it could be "reasonably deduced" that Massachusetts law did require a parent to provide medical attendance should a child's physical condition require it. Next, Judge Hudson emphasized that conviction for manslaughter in Massacusetts required the jury to determine that Dorothy Sheridan's behavior had not been merely negligent but rather "wanton or reckless," which Hudson further defined as an "indifference to, or a disregard of probable consequences" to Lisa's life. The jury returned a verdict of guilty, and Judge Hudson sentenced Sheridan to five years' probation. Jury members later told a reporter for the *Cape Cod News* that their deliberations had included parsing the meaning of the phrase "proper physical care." One juror said he found it disturbing the defense never indicated Sheridan had provided any form of physical care to Lisa at all, other than feeding her, during her extended illness. There had been heated discussion around the question of whether the tenets of Dorothy Sheridan's faith actually required her to ignore Lisa's physical needs. Unimpressed by the testimony concerning the respectability of Christian Science, they had been more interested in a statement made by David Sleeper, manager of the church's Committees on Publication, who had asserted that the decision to seek medical attendance rested with the individual church member. Ultimately, members of the jury determined that Dorothy Sheridan had been aware her daughter was seriously ill but made a conscious choice to deny her medical attention, a decision that had disregarded the probable consequences to Lisa's life.[12]

Unlike the trial of Merrill and Clara Reed over sixty years previously, the jury in the Sheridan case had been unwilling to consider metaphysical and medical treatment as equivalent responses to a child's serious illness. "A child sick for three weeks who doesn't have a doctor isn't being given 'sufficient physical care,' no matter which way you look at it," one juror later said. Proper physical care, in other words, had come to mean calling a physician when a child appeared to be seriously ill. Historians have noted that, in the era of the post-World War II "baby boom" physicians, particularly pediatricians, rose to unprecedented prominence as authoritative voices in child-rearing. Pediatrics had moved away from its early associations with hospitals and dispensaries serving poor and working-class neighborhoods in major cities to become one of the fastest-growing specialties among private practitioners; at the time Dorothy Sheridan was tried for manslaughter well over twelve thousand physicians in the United States limited their practice exclusively to children's health care. Benjamin Spock's *The Common Sense Book of Baby and Child Care*, which made its debut in 1946, became one of the best-selling books in American history. Spock, who was a 1927 graduate of Columbia University's College of Physicians and Surgeons, wrote in a tone that was reassuring and engaging rather than distant and clinical, reaffirming the notion that parents and physicians were partners in the scientific supervision of children's health. The text also addressed psychological concepts of personality development, introducing a new and complex dimension to child-rearing that intensified the level of scrutiny which parents, particularly mothers, were expected to devote to their children and, in turn, creating yet more demand for the services of pediatric specialists. But even households without a copy of *Baby and Child Care* on their bookshelves were routinely exposed to scientifically based information pertaining to children's health care. Expert medical advice filled the pages of newspapers and mass-market magazines and penetrated parents' consciousness via radio broadcasts and television shows. Given pediatricians' omnipresence in American life, by the 1960s it had become a commonsense notion that modern parenting required at least a basic familiarity with the latest medical thinking.[13]

But pediatricians were prepared to do more. In 1962 a seminal article published in the *Journal of the American Medical Association* launched a "pediatric reawakening" to the problem of child abuse, a domain previously dominated by social reformers working under the auspices of anti-cruelty organizations. In "The Battered Child Syndrome" authors C. Henry Kempe, Frederic N. Silverman, and Brandt F. Steel explained that x-ray technology had made it possible for physicians to identify distinctive types of bone fractures caused by the violent pulling or twisting of a child's arm or leg. These characteristic fractures visibly differed from the injuries children typically experienced during normal play activities. Thus x-ray machines, used in hospitals since the 1930s, were now extending physicians' gaze beneath the surface of children's bodies, providing a powerful new tool for those trained in the specialty of radiology to recognize signs of physical abuse. The authors concluded their paper with a professional call to arms, insisting that "physicians have a duty and responsibility to the child to require a full evaluation of the problem and to guarantee that no expected repetition of trauma will be permitted to occur." The widely-discussed article led to an upswell of support for the passage of new legislation requiring professionals who had regular contact with children, including medical practitioners, to report suspected abuse cases to child protection authorities. Five years after the publication of "The Battered Child Syndrome" forty-five states had enacted such mandated reporter laws.[14]

Nation-wide attention to the issue of child abuse featured physicians on the front lines of advancing children's physical welfare at a time when child-rearing itself had become substantially medicalized. Supporters of spiritual healing therefore worried that, despite the existing network of religious exemptions already in place and the Supreme Court's willingness to extend constitutional protections to religious practices as well as beliefs, the rights of parents to reject medical treatment for their children remained vulnerable to attack. One line of defense was to seek exemptions from the compulsory vaccination laws that had burgeoned during the polio scare of the 1950s. After the initial enthusiasm that greeted the Salk vaccine a proliferation of lawsuits were filed against drug manufacturers and governmental agencies by individuals claiming vaccine-related injuries. Although most of the lawsuits had been dismissed, a number had in fact been decided in favor of the victims, serving as a potent reminder to the public that immunization carried risks as well as rewards. Lingering medical uncertainties lent support to the notion that parents must be left alone to decide what was best for their children's health care. For Christian Scientists particularly, Dorothy Sheridan's manslaughter conviction made it clear that church members could find themselves convicted of serious crimes by juries who were unfamiliar with, or even hostile to, Mary Baker

Eddy's metaphysical paradigm explaining sickness and healing. "No jury is competent to judge the efficacy of Christian Science," David Sleeper, manager of the Committees on Publication, had declared following Sheridan's conviction. A second line of defense therefore was to secure specific statutory exemptions for religious healing within states' child endangerment laws. Church lobbyists in Massachusetts had already secured an exemption from compulsory school vaccination programs some months prior to Dorothy Sheridan's trial in 1967. They next turned their attention to the passage of legislation to establish once and for all that "proper physical care" included caring for sick or injured children using spiritual means. Entitled "A Bill Defining Proper Physical Care Under Laws Relating to the Care of Children by Parents," the bill that eventually cleared the statehouse read:

> A child shall not be deemed to be neglected or lack proper physical care for the sole reason that he is being provided remedial treatment by spiritual means alone in accordance with the tenets and practices of a recognized church or religious denomination by a duly-accredited practitioner thereof.

After some delay, in 1971 Massachusetts governor Francis Sargent signed the bill into law. A major challenge faced by the law's supporters had been crafting language that, while protecting healing practices that were particular to Christian Science, avoided the constitutional quagmire that would result if state law privileged one religion over others. In an unrelated case the state's high court had recently ruled that exemptions specific to particular religions violated the First Amendment's establishment clause. While it did not mention Christian Science by name, the bill's final version included the phrase "duly-accredited practitioner," a clear reference to the church's unique practice of certifying its own healers. Although both the American Medical Association and the Massachusetts Medical Society had charged that the new law sanctioned the physical suffering of children by allowing illness and injury to go untreated, most legislators had found it too politically risky to appear to deny the healing power of prayer.[15]

Meanwhile, outside of Massachusetts, momentum continued for elevating the problem of child abuse to the level of a national crisis. A watershed moment came in 1974 when Congress passed the Child Abuse Prevention and Treatment Act (CAPTA). Introduced by Senator Walter Mondale of Minnesota, CAPTA made available more than eighty-five million dollars to support the creation of new state-level programs. It set national standards for placing children removed from abusive homes into protective custody and also established a database for the purpose of collecting information about the nature and extent of the problem. The administration of this large and complex law was assigned to the Department of Health, Education and Welfare (HEW) which then had the responsibility of generating rules for its implementation. At this point a religious healing exemption, although not a part of the original CAPTA bill, appeared in the HEW regulations. While the precise explanation for the exemption's appearance remains unclear (authors disagree about the level of involvement Christian Scientists in the presidential administration of Richard M. Nixon might have had in its inclusion), the new regulation's language did clearly echo that of religious exemptions already in place in many states:

> A parent or guardian legitimately practicing his religious beliefs who thereby does not provide specified medical treatment for a child, for that reason alone shall not be considered a negligent parent or guardian; However such an exception shall not preclude a court from ordering that medical services be provided to the child, where his health requires it.[16]

Regardless of the exemption's murky origins this much was clear: Under CAPTA's administrative structure states must comply with HEW regulations in order to receive federal funding. As a result, states that did not already carve out religious exemptions in their child abuse and neglect laws now scrambled to enact them. Several statutes prohibited mandated reporters from alerting authorities when parents withheld medical care for their children on religious grounds. Twenty states went further, adding religious exemptions to their criminal codes defining manslaughter and homicide. Responding to objections from medical and children's rights organizations, in 1983 HEW changed course and rescinded its rule. Once enacted, however, laws can be extremely difficult to repeal and, what is more, the general public may have been unaware that religious exemptions had found their way into child endangerment laws that had been on the books since the late nineteenth century. Through the Committees on Publication the Christian Science church continued to disseminate its message supporting religious liberty as a core American value deserving of such legal protections. It also warned that repealing religious exemptions now set in place rendered all Christians vulnerable to discrimination merely for raising their children in accordance with their faith. "Our citizens don't want the legislature making sweeping judgments as to the inapplicability of serious Christianity in our time," the *Christian Science Sentinel* asserted in 1985.

"This is the kind of social control and curbing of valued freedoms characteristic of very different forms of government from our own." Invoking fears of totalitarian repression no doubt resonated with many Americans who had grown accustomed to strident anticommunist political rhetoric by the end of the Cold War. Despite HEW's reversal, the majority of states retained their exemptions.[17]

The consequences for children were soon enough apparent. In 1998, the journal *Pediatrics* reported that, between 1975 and 1995, 172 fatalities had occurred in the United States among children whose parents belonged to various faith-healing religions; forty-three cases had resulted in parents' criminal prosecution. While Christian Scientists had the highest public profile among the religions represented in the survey, several small and relatively unknown sects were also represented in the data. The General Assemblies and Church of the First Born, a Pentecostal church that had been formed in the early twentieth century, was associated with the deaths of at least two dozen children over a period of thirty years. Echoing John Alexander Dowie's Christian Catholic Church, members of the Church of the First Born eschewed mainstream medicine and relied exclusively on prayer and anointing with oil in healing illness and injury. The report's authors were Seth Asser, a pediatrician, and Rita Swan, a former Christian Scientist who, along with her husband Douglas, co-founded a non-profit group called Children's Healthcare is a Legal Duty (CHILD) following the death of their son in 1977. When sixteen-month-old Matthew fell ill the Swans had sought care from two different Christian Science practitioners. After a horrendous week watching his condition rapidly deteriorate and realizing he was in agonizing pain, the Swans finally brought Matthew to a hospital in Detroit, Michigan. Physicians diagnosed bacterial meningitis, an extremely dangerous disease that is also highly contagious. If caught at an early stage bacterial meningitis can be successfully treated with massive doses of antibiotics. By the time the Swans arrived at the hospital, however, it was too late and the child died several days later. Because they were protected by Michigan's religious exemptions, neither Matthew's parents nor the church practitioners who had attended his case faced criminal charges. Initially the Swans responded to the loss of their son by seeking reforms in the church's by-laws which, as had been the case in Mary Baker Eddy's time, prohibited certified healers from attending children who were also being treated by mainstream medical practitioners. When the Swans' efforts were rebuffed by church officials they made the difficult decision to abandon their religion and seek change by other means.[18]

The Swans took a highly unusual step: They pursued a wrongful death lawsuit against the Christian Science church and both of the practitioners they had engaged during Matthew's illness. It was the first such suit ever filed in the United States. The church responded with a motion for summary judgment, pointing out that Michigan's exemptions for spiritual healing practices rendered the Swans' lawsuit moot. The trial court granted the church's motion and, although the Swans filed an appeal, the case went no further. While the lawsuit's failure was a severe personal loss to the Swans, the legal proceeding did serve to reveal the immense gap that had grown between Mary Baker Eddy's healing precepts, originally laid out in 1875, and the range of scientific medical practices and treatments that were available to sick children more than a century later. In their depositions the two church practitioners testified that they had no knowledge of regular medicine and stressed that the church prohibited mixing spiritual treatment with *materia medica*. One healer explained her own commitment to avoiding all discussions of medical matters, going so far as to turn off radio and television programs whenever topics concerning health care arose. Neither healer was capable of recognizing a case of bacterial meningitis and in fact both had responded to the Swans' increasingly frantic questions by denying that the boy was ill at all, reminding the troubled parents that it was their own fears that posed the true danger to Matthew's well-being. The church practitioners were unaware of, and indeed uninterested in, the highly contagious nature of bacterial meningitis. Neither had reported the case to public health authorities, nor did they report the death of a second child from the same cause that had occurred just five blocks from the Swans' home. Perhaps seeking to demonstrate that Matthew was not really ill, one practitioner had encouraged Rita to allow him to play with his older sister. The little boy's death was not, in the practitioners' view, an indication that the church's healing system had failed. The church in fact did not record, or even acknowledge, the death of any child that occurred under the care of its certified practitioners.[19]

The Swans' lawsuit initiated a twenty-year period in which Christian Science healing practices faced a degree of public scrutiny unmatched since the early twentieth century. The Swans' efforts to make the public aware of the risks religious exemptions posed to children through their organization CHILD brought widespread attention to the issue. A series of criminal prosecutions of Christian Scientist parents took place in several different states when children, ranging in age from two to thirteen years, died without receiving medical attendance. Church members refer to these trials collectively as "the child cases." Drawing general conclusions about this period presents challenges given that the facts in each case varied and the specific charges differed from state to state. But, even with these caveats, the potentially grave consequences to children when states exempted religious practices in their child abuse and neglect laws were clearly evident. During the trials physicians testified that the causes of death, which included juvenile diabetes and bacterial meningitis as well as a bowel obstruction and a cancerous tumor of the leg, had been treatable conditions. Although medicine had still not become an exact science, it was possible to determine with a high degree of probability that each child's life would have been spared with timely intervention. Second, the trials revealed a clear disjuncture between the experiences of the victims and the priorities of the legal system. Trial juries, confronted with graphic testimony of the intense and prolonged suffering that the children had endured before their deaths, were willing to convict parents of serious crimes, including reckless conduct and manslaughter. But jury verdicts were often overturned, or sentences reduced, by appellate judges who interpreted religious exemptions as broad protections for parents' refusal to seek medical attention. Finally, the "child cases" revealed that many states had created a legal quagmire in which religious exemptions in abuse and neglect laws protected parents' choice to withhold medical care from an ailing child but the states' criminal codes punished the same decision if a child died.[20]

The problem was well illustrated in 1984 when the State of California filed both child endangerment and manslaughter charges against Laurie Walker in the death of her four-year-old daughter Shauntay. A Christian Scientist, Walker had treated the child exclusively with prayer for two weeks before she succumbed to bacterial meningitis. Legal complications arose because, in order to bring the state in compliance with CAPTA, the legislature had amended its 1872 child endangerment law to specify that treatment through "prayer alone in accordance with the tenets and practices of a recognized church or religious denomination," fell under the category of "other remedial care" and thus could not be construed as medical neglect. Attorneys for Walker filed a motion to stay the prosecution, arguing that California's exemption for spiritual healing precluded holding her criminally liable in her daughter's death. The state's supreme court denied the motion, however, determining that the legislature had not intended to provide an affirmative defense to manslaughter when it added the religious exemption to its child endangerment law; legislators had merely "remained silent" on that issue. Despite the court's green light to proceed in prosecuting the case, the Sacramento district attorney allowed Walker to plead guilty in return for receiving a relatively light sentence of five years' probation, community service, and a fine of three hundred dollars.[21]

As the twentieth century closed a significant backlash had mounted against what many Americans believed to be excessive governmental intrusion into parental prerogatives that had taken place in recent decades, represented most emblematically by the federal CAPTA law. "Parental rights" referendums began to appear on a number of state ballots. Although the initiatives did not reference religious liberty directly, Christian groups such as Of the People of Arlington, Virginia were heavily involved in campaigning for their support. "By restoring traditional parental authority," advocates argued, "the integrity and solidarity of the family unit is protected against intrusive outside forces. Parents know what is in the best interest of their children and families. Therefore, they should have constitutional protection to direct and control their children's lives until the children become adults." Thus the new wave of parental rights referendums both reflected and built upon the claims that had been previously advanced by backers of religious exemptions in child abuse and neglect laws. In 1995 the Parental Rights and Responsibilities Act was enacted by Congress with the aim of establishing higher barriers to intervention by state police and child protective services. Included among the parental rights the new federal law expressly sought to protect was the right to make health care decisions "unless those decisions resulted in a danger to the life of a child."[22]

By the mid-1990s controversies over religious exemptions in child neglect laws had also caught the attention of legal scholars.[23] Among the most outspoken critics of the exemptions was law professor James G. Dwyer. In 1997 Dwyer offered an extensive critique of the tendency, among judges and legal commentators alike, to consider the issue as a matter of competing constitutional interests between groups of adults. Debates about compulsory vaccination, for example, centered on the fact that states afforded protections to some parents on the basis of their religious affiliations but did not extend the same protections to parents who objected on secular grounds. For Dwyer such debates missed the essential point, for the real problem was that states were denying children equal treatment under the law, a requirement of the U. S. Constitution's Fourteenth Amendment. Dwyer's reframing of the issue rested on the premise that *all* children shared an interest in having their medical needs met and, what is more, well-established legal precedent permitted states to compel parents to provide medical attendance in cases of serious illness or injury. The introduction of religious exemptions in child neglect statutes, however, had created a state of affairs in which courts were required to balance *some* children's interests in accessing medical care against the religious preferences of their parents. Dwyer argued that such a balancing test was uniquely and unfairly demanded of children. "Courts would never consider the religious views of other persons as a justification for the state denying benefits to a particular group of adults," he insisted. The claim of equal protection, by contrast, would "impose upon the state the burden of showing that it (and not just the parents) has a sufficiently strong interest in denying protection to the child"—protection well established in the state's *parens patriae* role. Seconding Dwyer's call for change, other scholars stressed that shifting the legal focus to all children's right to the equal protection of the law avoided entangling courts in the constitutionally risky business of examining and evaluating whether specific religions' spiritual healing practices qualified as medical attendance or proper physical care. Still others pointed out that, while state and federal statutes permitted courts to intervene in parental decisions when cases involved extreme medical necessity, the definition of "medical necessity" itself remained unhelpfully vague. Was intervention permissible only when a child's life was deemed to be in danger? Or did it extend to cases in which the risk was not death but rather permanent injury or disability? Did assuaging physical pain and suffering constitute a medical necessity? Marci A. Hamilton, a law professor and leading advocate for children's rights in the United States, bluntly disparaged all such judicial balancing efforts as a "zero sum game" in which "it is the children who are sacrificed, instead of the religious conduct."[24]

Left largely unaddressed in the discourses surrounding religious-based medical neglect and children's right to equal treatment under the law was the question of whether any child—healthy or sick—was entitled to health care in the United States. As Sydney Halpern perceptively observed, the medical specialty of pediatrics had been the product of a "social movement much broader than medicine," a child welfare crusade that had placed children's well-being at the center of a comprehensive vision of social progress. The apex of the progressive child welfare movement had been the establishment of the United States Children's Bureau in 1912. The Bureau, in turn, was instrumental in Congress's passage of the Sheppard-Towner Act nine years later. Sheppard-Towner granted federal funds to states for the development of maternal and infant health education programs, an issue prioritized by child welfare advocates who were troubled that rates of infant and maternal mortality remained stubbornly high at a time when deaths due to other diseases were declining. The identification of bacteria as the culprit behind the long-dreaded cholera infantum and other notorious killers, coupled with the early successes of antitoxin in preventing diphtheria deaths, generated considerable enthusiasm for disseminating the benefits of medical science far beyond the laboratory and advanced the notion that all children deserved to benefit from the new discoveries. But, despite tangible and significant achievements in improving children's life-chances, the early twentieth-century child welfare movement did not ultimately succeed in overcoming Americans' deep-seated racial and class divisions sufficiently to convince them that the medical care of children constituted a shared national interest. Instead, enthusiasm for the scientific medical care of children was channeled into a private-sector demand for the professional services of physicians. As regular medical practitioners became the foremost social authorities on child-rearing, they pushed aside social reformers' comprehensive vision of children's well-being. Activist physicians in the American Medical Association and state medical societies directly challenged the expertise of non-scientist reformers in the child welfare movement. With support from politically organized physicians Congress allowed the Sheppard-Tower Act to expire without renewal in 1929; the Children's Bureau's was dismantled as an administrative agency less than twenty years later. By mid-century pediatricians had left the dispensary and well-baby clinic en masse and assumed new roles as supervising children's health in private practice. When the subject of child abuse and neglect reappeared in the 1960s it was framed within a context of doctors' authority and professional expertise rather than a comprehensive vision of state-supported social reforms intended to improve the physical well-being of all children.[25]

At the end of the twentieth century, a broad spectrum of the American public agreed that proper parenting required at least some familiarity with the latest scientific information concerning children's health and cooperation with the professionals who practiced medicine. The outcomes of criminal trials indicated juries' willingness to punish individual parents who failed to provide their children with mainstream medical attendance, even if such choices were informed by the tenets of the parents' faith. But, even as the nation pressed forward into the new millennium, Americans remained less certain that children's access to scientifically advanced medical care constituted a shared national interest. When the Affordable Care Act took effect in 2014, it included special exemptions for those whose "sincerely held religious beliefs against medical health care" precluded them from buying health insurance, for themselves or their children, as mandated by the law. As long as adults' liberty to deny medical care to children remains enshrined within American law, children whose physical well-being, and indeed their very lives, may depend upon the science of the age remain vulnerable.[26]

## NOTES

1. *Bradley v. State* 79 Fla 651, 1920.
2. *Bradley v. State.*
3. James Colgrove, *State of Immunity: The Politics of Vaccination in Twentieth-Century America* (Berkeley: University of California Press, 2006), 82–86; Sydney A. Halpern, *American Pediatrics: The Social Dynamics of Professionalism, 1880–1980* (Berkeley: University of California Press, 1988), 80–81; Suellen Hoy, *Chasing Dirt: The American Pursuit of Cleanliness* (New York: Oxford University Press, 1995); Carolyn Fraser, *God's Perfect Child: Living and Dying in the Christian Science Church* (New York: Henry Holt, 1999), 203.
4. "Smallpox in Zion Admitted *God's Perfect Child: Living and Dying in the Christian Science Church*," *Chicago Daily Tribune* (August 9, 1902): 3; Stephen Gottschalk, *Rolling Away the Stone: Mary Baker Eddy's Challenge to Materialism* (Bloomington: Indiana University Press, 2006), 350–351.
5. Young, "Defending Child Medical Neglect," 271–277; Fraser, *God's Perfect Child*, 272–279; Shawn Francis Peters, *When Prayer Fails: Faith Healing, Children, and the Law* (Oxford: Oxford University Press, 2008), 108.
6. *Pierce v. Society of Sisters* 268 U.S. 510 (1925); *Prince v. Massachusetts* 321 U.S. 158 (1944).
7. *Sherbert v. Verner* 374 U.S. 398 (1963); *Wisconsin v. Yoder* 406 U.S. 25 (1972).
8. Colgrove, *State of Immunity*, 114–116; Naomi Rogers, *Dirt and Disease: Polio Before FDR* (New Brunswick: Rutgers University Press, 1992; "2 Take Stand in Fight Over Polio Vaccine," *Chicago Daily Tribune* (April 18, 1957): 10.
9. Fraser, *God's Perfect Child*, 277–279; Robert L. Trescher and Thomas N. O'Neill, Jr., "Medical Care for Dependent Children: Manslaughter Liability of the Christian Scientist," *University of Pennsylvania Law Review*, Volume 109, Number 2 (December 1960): 203–217.
10. Fraser, *God's Perfect Child*, 279–282.
11. Leo Damore covered Dorothy Sheridan's trial for the *Cape Cod News* and subsequently wrote a book on the case. *The "Crime" of Dorothy Sheridan* (Westminster, MD: Arbor House, 1978), 209–235.

12. Damore concluded that, in refusing to grant validity to Christian Science metaphysical teachings, the jury had also found the church guilty in Lisa Sheridan's death. *The "Crime" of Dorothy Sheridan*, 274–283.

13. Damore, *The "Crime" of Dorothy Sheridan*, 281; Halpern, *American Pediatrics*, 82–83; Rima D. Apple, *Perfect Motherhood: Science and Childrearing in America* (New Brunswick: Rutgers University Press, 2005).

14. C. Henry Kempe, Frederic N. Silverman, and Brandt F. Steele et al., "The Battered Child Syndrome," *Journal of the American Medical Association*, Volume 181, Number 1 (1962): 17–24; Judith Sealander, *The Failed Century of the Child: Governing America's Young in the Twentieth Century* (New York: Cambridge University Press, 2003), 61–64. C. Henry Kempe went on to become a leading national figure bringing attention to the problem of child sexual abuse. Hughes Evans, "The Discovery of Child Sexual Abuse in America." In Alexandra Minna Stern and Howard Markel, editors, *Formative Years: Children's Health in the United States 1880–1920* (Ann Arbor: University of Michigan Press, 2004), 233–259.

15. Colgrove, *State of Immunity*, 186–217; Fraser, *God's Perfect Child*, 282–283; Damore, *The "Crime" of Dorothy Sheridan*, 307–314; Rennie B. Schoepflin, *Christian Science on Trial: Religious Healing in America* (Baltimore: Johns Hopkins University Press, 2003), 202; N. E. Talbot, "The Position of the Christian Science Church," *New England Journal of Medicine*, Volume 309 (1983): 1641–1644.

16. Peters, *When Prayer Fails*, 116–117. Religious scholar Ronald B. Flowers reported finding no documentary evidence that Christian Scientists had influenced HEW's introduction of the religious exemption. "Withholding Medical Care for Religious Reasons," *Journal of Religion and Health*, Volume 23, Number 4 (Winter 1984): 268–282. Rita Swan argued that two Christian Scientists who were powerful members of president Richard M. Nixon's administration, H. R. Haldeman and John Erlichman, may have been responsible. Caroline Fraser shared Swan's view, also noting the high degree of involvement that Haldeman and Erlichman had in securing a copyright extension for *Science and Health with Key to the Scriptures*, which was about to enter the public domain in 1971. *God's Perfect Child*, 240–243. More recently physician Paul A. Offit discussed the involvement of Haldeman and Erlichman in the religious exemption's appearance in HEW regulations. *Bad Faith: When Religious Belief Undermines Modern Medicine* (New York: Basic Books, 2015), 170–171.

17. Rita Swan, "On Statutes Depriving a Class of Children of Rights to Medical Care: Can This Discrimination Be Litigated? *Quinnipiac Health Law Journal*, Volume 2, Number 73 (1998): 73–96; Shirley Darby Howell, "Religious Treatment Exemption Statutes: Betrayest Thou Me with a Statute?" *St. Mary's Law Review on Minority Issues*, Volume 14 (Spring 2012): 946–984; Gregory Engle, "Towards a New Lens of Analysis: The

History and Future of Religious Exemptions to Child Neglect Statutes," *Richmond Journal of Law and the Public Interest*, Volume 14, Number 2 (2015): 375–399; Young, "Christian Science Persuasive Rhetoric," 283.

18. Peters, *When Prayer Fails*, 175–192; Seth M. Asser and Rita Swan, "Child Fatalities from Religious-Motivated Medical Neglect," *Pediatrics*, Volume 101, Number 4 (April 1998): 625–629. Subsequent to the publication of this report Swan identified another seven cases, bringing the number of criminal prosecutions to fifty. "On Statutes Depriving a Class of Children to Medical Care," 78.

19. The information from the depositions in the Swans' lawsuit, augmented by personal interviews with Rita Swan, appears in Fraser, *God's Perfect Child*, 286–296.

20. Alan Rogers, *The Child Cases: How America's Religious Exemption Laws Harm Children* (Amherst: University of Massachusetts Press, 2014), 1–20; Peters, *When Prayer Fails*, 116–117.

21. *Walker v. Superior Court*, 47 Cal.3d 112, 1988.

22. Linda L. Lane, "The Parental Rights Movement," *University of Colorado Law Review* Volume 69 (1998): 825–832; Judith Sealander, *The Failed Century of the Child*, 79–84.

23. Legal scholarship on religious exemptions was voluminous in the period ca. 1995–2005. See for example: Larry May, "Challenging Medical Authority: The Refusal of Treatment by Christian Scientists," *The Hastings Center Report*, Volume 25, Number 1 (January–February 1995): 15–21; Richard T. De George, Margaret Pabst Battin, H. Hamner Hill, Kenneth Kipnis, and Larry May, "Christian Science's Right to Refuse," *The Hastings Center Report*, Volume 25, Number 4 (July–August 1995): 2–3; Elizabeth Lingle, "Treating Children by Faith: Colliding Constitutional Issues," *Journal of Legal Medicine*, Volume 17 (June 1996): 301–330; Lauren A. Greenberg, "In God We Trust: Faith Healing Subject to Liability," *Journal of Contemporary Health Law and Policy*, Volume 14 (Spring 1998): 451–476; Janna C. Merrick, "Spiritual Healing, Sick Kids, and the Law: Inequities in the American Health Care System," *American Journal of Law and Medicine*, Volume 29 (2003): 269–299; Allison Ciullo, "Prosecution Without Persecution: The Inability of Courts to Recognize Christian Science Healing and a Shift Towards Legislative Action," *New England Law Review* Volume 43 (Fall 2007): 156–194. A reference guide to earlier publications is Elena M. Kondos, "The Law and Christian Science Healing for Children: A Pathfinder," *Legal Reference Services Quarterly*, Volume 12, Number 1 (1992): 5–72.

24. James G. Dwyer, "The Children We Abandon: Religious Exemptions to Child Welfare and Education Laws As Denials of Equal Protection to Children of Religious Objectors," *North Carolina Law Review* Volume

74 (1996): 1321–1471; Gregory Engle, "Towards a New Lens of Analysis: The History and Future of Religious Exemptions to Child Neglect Statutes," *Richmond Journal of Law and the Public Interest*, Volume 14, Number 2 (2015): 375–399; Robert H. Mnookin and D. Kelly Weisberg, *Child, Family, and State: Problems and Materials on Children in the Law* (New York: Aspen Publishers, 2000), 599–655; Marci A. Hamilton, *God vs. the Gavel: Religion and the Rule of Law* (New York: Cambridge University Press, 2005), 13.

25. Halpern, *American Pediatrics*, 106; On divisions and shortcomings in the progressive child welfare movement and their longer-term consequences see Katharine S. Bullard, *Civilizing the Child: Discourses of Race, Nation, and Child Welfare in America* (Lanham, MD: Lexington Books, 2014) and Kriste Lindenmeyer, *"A Right to Childhood": The U.S. Children's Bureau and Child Welfare, 1912–1946* (Urbana: University of Illinois Press, 1997).

26. Offitt, *Bad Faith*, 192.

# Bibliography

## Manuscript Collections

Records of the Massachusetts Metaphysical College, The Mary Baker Eddy Library, Boston, MA.
Cook County Medical Examiner's Reports, Illinois Regional Archives Depository, Northeastern Illinois University, Chicago, IL.

## Newspapers and Periodicals

*A Voice from Zion*
*Boston Evening Herald*
*Chicago Daily Herald*
*Chicago Daily Tribune*
*Chicago Inter-Ocean*
*Chicago Record-Herald*
*Christian Advocate*
*Christian Science Journal*
*Illinois Medical Journal*
*Journal of the American Medical Association*
*Leaves of Healing*
*Los Angeles Times*
*New York Evening Journal*
*New York Herald*

© The Editor(s) (if applicable) and The Author(s), under exclusive license to Springer Nature Switzerland AG 2019
L. Curry, *Religion, Law, and the Medical Neglect of Children in the United States, 1870–2000*, Palgrave Studies in the History of Childhood, https://doi.org/10.1007/978-3-030-24689-1

*New York Medical Journal*
*New York Times*
*New York Tribune*
*Quincy Daily Journal*
*Quincy Daily Whig*
*St. Louis Republic*
*The World*

## PRIMARY SOURCES

"A Bogus Medical College—The Massachusetts Bellevue," *Annual Report of the Illinois State Board of Health 1880*. Springfield, IL: H.W. Rocker, 1881.

Baker, Josephine. *Fighting for Life*. Reprinted by the New York Review of Books, 2013.

Beck, John R. *Essays on Infant Therapeutics*. New York: W.E. Dean, 1849.

Biggs, Hermann M. "The New Treatment of Diphtheria," *McClure's Magazine*, Volume IV, Number 4 (March 1895): 360–364.

Blackstone, William. *Commentaries on the Laws of England*, Volume 1. Reprinted in Robert H. Mnookin and D. Kelly Weisberg, editors, *Child, Family, and State*. Frederick, MD: Aspen Publishers, 2000.

Brace, Charles Loring. *The Races of the Old World: A Manual of Ethnology*. New York: Charles Scribner, 1863.

———. *The Dangerous Classes and Twenty Years Work Among Them*. Third edition. New York: Wynkoop and Hallenbeck, 1880.

Buchan, William. *Domestic Medicine, or A Treatise for the Cure and Prevention of Diseases, By Regimen and Simple Medicines*. Halifax: Milner and Sowerby, 1859.

———. *Domestic Medicine; or The Family Physician*. Philadelphia: John Dunlap, 1772. Reprinted Ann Arbor: Text Creation Partnership, 2008.

Cadogan, William. *An Essay Upon Nursing and the Management of Children From Their Birth to Three Years of Age*. London: Jay Roberts, 1748.

Cather, Willa, and Georgine Milmine. *The Life of Mary Baker G. Eddy and the History of Christian Science*. New York: Doubleday, Page and Company, 1909.

*The Chicago Daily News Almanac and Year Book*. Chicago: Chicago Daily News Company, 1902.

*Christian Science and Legislation*. Boston, MA: The Christian Science Publishing Company, 1906.

Condie, David Francis. *A Practical Treatise on the Diseases of Children*. Second edition. Philadelphia: Lea and Blanchard, 1847.

"Construction of a Statute. *State v. Mylod* 40 Atl. Rep. (R.I.) 753," *The Yale Law Journal*, Volume 8, Number 1 (October 1898): 57.

*Criminal Law and Procedure of California*. Los Angeles: Charles W. Balm Company, 1902.

Dewees, William Potts. *A Treatise on the Physical and Medical Treatment of Children*. Philadelphia: H. C. Carey and I. Lea, 1825.

Dowie, John Alexander Dowie. *Zion's Holy War Against the Hosts of Hell in Chicago*. Chicago: Zion Publishing House, 1900.

———. *Doctors, Drugs, and Devils*. Zion, IL: Zion Publishing House, 1901.

Eberle, John. *A Treatise on the Diseases and Physical Education of Children*. Cincinnati, OH: Corey and Fairbank, 1833.

Eddy, Mary Baker (Glover). *Science and Health with Key to the Scriptures*. Boston: Christian Scientist Publishing Company, 1875.

———. *Science and Health with Key to the Scriptures*. Third edition revised. Lynn, MA: Dr. Asa G. Eddy, 1881.

———. *Science and Health with Key to the Scriptures*. Fortieth edition. Boston: Mary Baker G. Eddy, 1889.

———. *Retrospection and Introspection*. Boston: Trustees of the First Church of Christ, Scientist, 1891.

———. *Science and Health with Key to the Scriptures*. Seventy-seventh edition, revised. Boston: E. J. Foster Eddy, 1893.

———. *Science and Health with Key to the Scriptures*. Boston: Joseph A. Armstrong, 1902.

———. *Science and Health with Key to the Scriptures*. Boston: Trustees of the First Church of Christ, Scientist, 1906.

———. "Contagion." In *Miscellaneous Writings 1883–1896*. Boston: Trustees under the will of Mary Baker G. Eddy, 1924.

Evans, Warren Felt. *The New Age and Its Messenger*. Boston: T.H. Carter and Company, 1864.

Harlan, Rolvix. *John Alexander Dowie and the Christian Catholic Apostolic Church*. Evansville, WI: Press of Robert M. Antes, 1906.

Hertzler, Arthur E. *The Horse and Buggy Doctor*. New York: Harper and Brothers, 1938.

Holt, Luther Emmett. *The Diseases of Infancy and Childhood*. Second edition. New York: D. Appleton and Company, 1899.

Illinois State Board of Health. *Report on Medical Education and Official Register of Legally Qualified Physicians*. Springfield, IL: Illinois State Register, 1903.

Jacobi, Abraham. *Infant Diet*. Revised, Enlarged, and Adapted to Public Use by Mary Putnam Jacobi. New York: G.P. Putnam's Sons, 1874.

———. *A Treatise on Diphtheria*. New York: William Wood and Company, 1880.

———. "Address at the Twenty-Fifth Jubilee of the German Dispensary of New York." In A. Jacobi, editor, *Miscellaneous Addresses and Writings*, Volume VIII. New York: The Critic and Guide Company, 1909.

Kempe, C. Henry, Frederic N. Silverman, Brandt F. Steele, et al. "The Battered Child Syndrome," *Journal of the American Medical Association*, Volume 181, Number 1 (1962): 17–24.

Lindsay, Gordon, editor. *The Sermons of John Alexander Dowie*. Shreveport, LA: Voice of Healing Publishing, n.d.

Locke, John. *Some Thoughts Concerning Education*. London: Ward, Lock, and Company, 1693.

*The Los Angeles Case; The People Versus Merrill Reed et al*. Boston: The Christian Science Publishing Society, 1904.

Meigs, John Forsyth. *A Practical Treatise on the Diseases of Children*. Philadelphia: Lindsay and Blakiston, 1848.

National Congress of Mothers. *The Work and Words of the First National Congress of Mothers*. New York: D. Appleton, 1897.

National League for Medical Freedom. *The Facts About "Colliers'" Attack on the National League for Medical Freedom*. New York: National League for Medical Freedom, 1912.

O'Dwyer, Joseph. *Intubation in Croup and Other Acute and Chronic Forms of Stenosis of the Larynx*. New York: William Wood and Company, 1889.

Palmer, John McAuley, editor. *The Bench and Bar of Illinois: Historical and Reminiscent*, Volume 2. Chicago: The Lewis Publishing Company, 1899.

Park, William Hallock. "Diphtheria and Other Pseudomembranous Inflammations—A Clinical and Bacteriological Study," *New York Medical Record*, Volume 43, Number 6 (Winter 1893): 161–168.

———. "Diphtheria Antitoxine—Its Production," *McClure's Magazine*, Volume IV, Number 4 (March 1895): 365–369.

Purrington, William A. *A Review of Recent Legal Decisions Affecting Physicians, Dentists, Druggists and the Public Health*. New York: E.B. Treat and Company, 1899.

———. *Christian Science*. New York: E.B. Treat and Company, 1900.

Quimby, Phineas Parkhurst. "The Effect of Mind Upon Mind." In Horatio W. Dresser, editor, *The Quimby Manuscripts*. New York: The Julian Press, 1961a.

———. "The Treatment of a Child." In Horatio W. Dresser, editor, *The Quimby Manuscripts*. New York: The Julian Press, 1961b.

Reynolds, Arthur R. "Reminiscences of Ten Years as Commissioner of Health in Chicago, and Suggestions for the Future," *California State Journal of Medicine*, Volume VII, Number 6 (June 1909): 218–221.

Riis, Jacob. *The Children of the Poor*. New York: Charles Scribner's Sons, 1908.

Schouler, James. *A Treatise on the Law of Domestic Relations*. Boston: Little, Brown, and Company, 1870.

Sheldrake, Edna Sheldrake, editor. *The Personal Letters of John Alexander Dowie*. Zion, IL: Wilbur Glenn Voliva, 1912.

Smith, Job Lewis. *A Treatise on the Diseases of Infancy and Children*. Second edition. Philadelphia: Henry C. Lee, 1872.

Starr, Merritt, and Russell H. Curtis, editors. *Annotated Statutes of the State of Illinois*, Volume I. Chicago: Callahan and Company, 1885.

Talbot, N. E. "The Position of the Christian Science Church," *New England Journal of Medicine*, Volume 309 (1983): 1641–1644.
Twain, Mark. *Christian Science*. New York: Elibron Classics, 2006.

## LEGAL CASES

*Bennett v. Ware* 1908.
*Bradley v. State* 1920.
*Commonwealth v. Thomson* 1809.
*Dent v. State of West Virginia* 1889.
*Edward Cowley v. State of New York* 4 1881.
*Henrikka Bratsch v. The People* 1902.
*Jacobsen v. Massachusetts* 1905.
*New York v. J. Luther Pierson* 1903.
*Owens v. State* 6 1911.
*People v. Merrill Reed et al* 1902.
*People v. Quimby* 1906.
*Pierce v. Society of Sisters* 1925.
*Prince v. Massachusetts* 1944.
*Queen v. Wagstaffe* 1868.
*Reynolds v. United States* 1878.
*Sherbert v. Verner* 1963.
*State v. Blue Mountain Joe* 1889.
*State v. Buswell* 1894.
*State v. Joseph P. Gordon* 1902.
*State v. Mylod* 1898.
*Walker v. Superior Court* 1988.
*Wisconsin v. Yoder* 1972.

## SECONDARY SOURCES

Albanese, Catherine L. *A Republic of Mind and Spirit: A Cultural History of American Metaphysical Religion*. New Haven, CT: Yale University Press, 2007.
Apple, Rima D. *Perfect Motherhood: Science and Childrearing in America*. New Brunswick, NJ: Rutgers University Press, 2005.
Ashby, LeRoy. *Endangered Children: Dependency, Neglect, and Abuse in American History*. New York: Twayne Publishers, 1997.
Asser, Seth M., and Rita Swan. "Child Fatalities from Religious-Motivated Medical Neglect," *Pediatrics*, Volume 101, Number 4 (April 1998): 625–629.
Badaracco, Claire Hoertz. *Prescribing Faith: Medicine, Media, and Religion in American Culture*. Waco, TX: Baylor University Press, 2007.

Barnes, Linda L., and Susan S. Sered, editors. *Religion and Healing in America.* New York: Oxford University Press, 2005.

Benziman, Galia. *Narratives of Child Neglect in Romantic and Victorian Culture.* New York: Palgrave Macmillan, 2012.

Bonner, Thomas Neville. *Medicine in Chicago, 1850–1950.* Second edition. Urbana, IL: University of Illinois Press, 1991.

Braden, Charles S. *Spirits in Rebellion: The Rise and Development of New Thought.* University Park, TX: Southern Methodist University Press, 1963.

Brandon, Mark E. *States of Union: Families and Change in the American Constitutional Order.* Lawrence, KS: University Press of Kansas, 2013.

Brosco, Jeffrey P. "Weight Charts and Well Child Care: When the Pediatrician Became the Expert in Child Health." In Alexandra Minna Stern and Howard Markel, editors, *Formative Years: Children's Health in the United States, 1880–2000.* Ann Arbor, MI: University of Michigan Press, 2004, 91–120.

Brown, Kathleen M. *Foul Bodies: Cleanliness in Early America.* New Haven, CT: Yale University Press, 2007.

Bullard, Katharine S. *Civilizing the Child: Discourses of Race, Nation, and Child Welfare in America.* Lanham, MD: Lexington Books, 2014.

Calvert, Karen. *Children in the House: The Material Culture of Early Childhood, 1600–1900.* Boston: Northeastern University Press, 1992.

Cayleff, Susan E. *Nature's Path: A History of Naturopathic Healing in America.* Baltimore: Johns Hopkins University Press, 2016.

Cheney, Rose A. "Seasonal Aspects of Infant and Childhood Mortality: Philadelphia, 1865–1920," *Journal of Interdisciplinary History*, Volume 14, Number 3 (Winter 1984): 561–585.

CHILD USA. "Religious Exemptions to Medical Care of Sick Children (As of 2017)." https://www.childusa.org/medicalneglect/.

Cohen, Michael H. *Complementary & Alternative Medicine: Legal Boundaries and Regulatory Perspectives.* Baltimore: Johns Hopkins University Press, 1995.

Colgrove, James. *State of Immunity: The Politics of Vaccination in Twentieth-Century America.* Berkeley: University of California Press, 2006.

Cone, Thomas E., Jr. *History of American Pediatrics.* Boston: Little, Brown, and Company, 1979.

Cook, Philip L. *Zion City, Illinois.* Syracuse, NY: Syracuse University Press, 1996.

Costin, Lela B. "Unraveling the Mary Ellen Legend: Origins of the 'Cruelty' Movement," *Social Service Review*, Volume 65, Number 2 (June 1991): 203–223.

Crabtree, Adam. *From Mesmer to Freud: Magnetic Sleep and the Roots of Psychological Healing.* New Haven, CT: Yale University Press, 1993.

Cunningham, Hugh. *Children and Childhood in Western Society Since 1500.* Second edition. Harlow, UK: Pearson Education Limited, 2005.

Curry, Lynne. *Modern Mothers in the Heartland: Gender, Health, and Progress in Illinois, 1900–1930.* Columbus, OH: The Ohio State University Press.

Curtis, Heather D. *Faith in the Great Physician: Suffering and Divine Healing in American Culture, 1860–1900*. Baltimore: Johns Hopkins University Press, 2007.

Czerniawski, Amanda M. "From Average to Ideal: The Evolution of the Height and Weight Table in the United States, 1836–1943," *Social Science History*, Volume 31, Number 2 (Summer 2007): 273–296.

Damore, Leo. *The "Crime" of Dorothy Sheridan*. Westminster, MD: Arbor House, 1978.

Darnton, Robert. *Mesmerism and the End of the Enlightenment in France*. Revised edition. Cambridge, MA: Harvard University Press, 1986.

Davidovitch, Nadav. "Negotiating Dissent: Homeopathy and Anti-Vaccinationism at the Turn of the Twentieth Century." In Robert D. Johnston, editor, *The Politics of Healing: Histories of Alternative Healing in Twentieth-Century North America*. Abingdon, UK: Routledge, 2004.

Davis, David J., editor. *The History of Medical Practice in Illinois, Volume II, 1850–1900*. Chicago: Illinois State Medical Society, 1955.

DeLuzio, Crista. *Female Adolescence in American Scientific Thought, 1830–1930*. Baltimore: Johns Hopkins University Press, 2007.

Demaitre, Luke. *Medieval Medicine: The Art of Healing, from Head to Toe*. Santa Barbara, CA: Praeger, 2013.

Demos, John. *A Little Commonwealth: Family Life in Plymouth Colony*. Second edition. New York: Oxford University Press 2000.

Donegan, Jane B. *"Hydropathic Highway to Health": Women and Water-Cure in Antebellum America*. Santa Barbara, CA: Praeger, 1986.

Dowling, Harry F. *Fighting Infection: Conquests of the Twentieth Century*. Cambridge, MA: Harvard University Press, 1977.

Duane, Anna Mae. *Suffering Childhood in Early America: Violence, Race, and the Making of the Child Victim*. Athens: University of Georgia Press, 2010.

Duffy, John. *From Humors to Medical Science: A History of American Medicine*. Second edition. Urbana: University of Illinois Press, 1993.

Evans, Hughes. "The Discovery of Child Sexual Abuse in America." In Alexandra Minna Stern and Howard Markel, editors, *Formative Years: Children's Health in the United States 1880–1920*. Ann Arbor: University of Michigan Press, 2004, 233–259.

Fineman, Dorothy Albertson. "What Is Right for Children?" In Dorothy Albertson Fineman and Karen Worthington, editors, *What Is Right for Children? The Competing Paradigms of Religion and Human Rights*. Burlington, VT: Ashgate, 2009, 1–4.

Finger, Stanley. *Doctor Franklin's Medicine*. Philadelphia: University of Pennsylvania Press, 2006.

Fliegelman, Jay. *Prodigals and Pilgrims: The American Revolution Against Patriarchal Authority 1750–1800*. Cambridge: Cambridge University Press, 1982.

Flowers, Ronald B. "Withholding Medical Care for Religious Reasons," *Journal of Religion and Health*, Volume 23, Number 4 (Winter 1984): 268–282.

Foucault, Michel. *The Birth of the Clinic: An Archaeology of Medical Perception*. A. M. Sheridan Smith, translator. New York: Vintage Books, 1994.

Fraser, Caroline. *God's Perfect Child: Living and Dying in the Christian Science Church*. New York: Henry Holt 1999.

Fuller, Robert C. *Alternative Medicine and American Religious Life*. New York: Oxford University Press, 1989.

———. *The Body of Faith: A Biological History of Religion in America*. Chicago: University of Chicago Press, 2013.

Gandall, Keith. *The Virtues of the Vicious: Jacob Riis, Stephen Crane, and the Spectacle of the Slum*. New York: Oxford University Press, 1997.

Gear, Josephine. "The Baby's Picture: Woman as Image Maker in Small-Town America," *Feminist Studies*, Volume 13, Number 2 (Summer 1987): 419–442.

Gevitz, Norman, editor. *Other Healers: Unorthodox Medicine in America*. Baltimore: Johns Hopkins University Press, 1988.

———. "Christian Science Healing and the Health Care of Children," *Perspectives in Biology and Medicine*, Volume 34, Number 3 (Spring 1991): 421–438.

———. *The DOs: Osteopathic Medicine in America*. Second edition. Baltimore: Johns Hopkins University Press, 2004.

Gill, Gillian. *Mary Baker Eddy*. New York: Perseus Books, 1998.

Glenn, Myra C. *Campaigns Against Corporal Punishment: Prisoners, Sailors, Women, and Children in Antebellum America*. Albany, NY: State University of New York Press, 1984.

Gloege, Timothy E. W. "Faith Healing, Medical Regulation, and Public Religion in Progressive Era Chicago," *Religion and American Culture: A Journal of Interpretation*, Volume 23, Number 2 (Summer 2013): 185–231.

Golden, Janet, Richard A. Meckel, and Heather Munroe Prescott, editors. *Children and Youth in Sickness and in Health*. Westport, CT: Greenwood Press, 2004.

Gordon, Linda. *Heroes of Their Own Lives: The Politics and History of Family Violence*. New York: Penguin Books, 1988.

———. "The Perils of Innocence, or What's Wrong with Putting Children First," *Journal of the History of Children and Youth*, Volume 1, Number 3 (Fall 2008): 331–350.

Gottschalk, Stephen. *Rolling Away the Stone: Mary Baker Eddy's Challenge to Materialism*. Bloomington, IN: Indiana University Press, 2006.

Grossberg, Michael. *Governing the Hearth: Law and the Family in Nineteenth-Century America*. Chapel Hill, NC: University of North Carolina Press, 1985.

Haller, John S., Jr. *American Medicine in Transition 1840–1910*. Urbana, IL: University of Illinois Press, 1981.

Halpern, Sydney A. *American Pediatrics: The Social Dynamics of Professionalism, 1880–1980*. Berkeley, CA: University of California Press, 1988.

Hamilton, Marci A. *God vs. the Gavel: Religion and the Rule of Law.* New York: Cambridge University Press, 2005.

Hammonds, Evelynn Maxine. *Childhood's Deadly Scourge: The Campaign to Control Diphtheria in New York City, 1880–1930.* Baltimore: Johns Hopkins University Press, 1999.

Hardy, Anne. "Tracheotomy Versus Intubation: Surgical Intervention in Diphtheria in Europe and the United States, 1825–1930," *Bulletin of the History of Medicine*, Volume 66 (1992): 536–559.

Harrell, David Edwin, Jr. "Divine Healing in Modern American Protestantism." In Norman Gevitz, editor, *Other Healers: Unorthodox Medicine in America.* Baltimore: Johns Hopkins University Press, 1988, 215–227.

Hazen, Craig James. *The Village Enlightenment in America: Popular Religion and Science in the Nineteenth Century.* Urbana, IL: University of Illinois Press, 2000.

Heath, Alden H. "Apostle in Zion," *Journal of the Illinois State Historical Society*, Volume 70, Number 2 (May 1977): 98–113.

Herndon, Ruth Wallis. "'Proper' Magistrates and Masters: Binding Out Poor Children in Southern New England, 1720–1820." In Ruth Wallis Herndon and John E. Murray, editors, *Children Bound to Labor: The Pauper Apprentice System in Early America.* Ithaca, NY: Cornell University Press, 2009.

Hoffert, Sylvia. *Private Matters: American Attitudes Toward Childbearing and Infant Nurture in the Urban North, 1800–1860.* Urbana, IL: University of Illinois Press, 1989.

Hollenweger, Walter J. *The Pentecostals.* Minneapolis, MN: Augsburg Press, 1972.

Hoy, Suellen. *Chasing Dirt: The American Pursuit of Cleanliness.* New York: Oxford University Press, 1995.

Johnson, David A., and Humayun J. Chaudhry. *Medicine Licensing and Discipline in America.* Lanham, MD: Lexington Books, 2012.

Johnston, Robert D. *The Radical Middle Class: Populist Democracy and the Question of Capitalism in Progressive Era Portland, Oregon.* Princeton, NJ: Princeton University Press, 2003.

Judah, J. Stillson. *The History and Philosophy of Metaphysical Movements in America.* Louisville, KY: Westminster Press, 1967.

Lane, Linda L. "The Parental Rights Movement," *University of Colorado Law Review*, Volume 69 (1998): 825–832.

Lavender, Caroline F. *Cradle of Liberty: Race, the Child, and National Belonging from Thomas Jefferson to W. E. B. DuBois.* Durham, NC: Duke University Press, 2006.

Lears, T. J. Jackson. *No Place of Grace: Antimodernism and the Transformation of American Culture, 1880–1920.* New York: Pantheon Books, 1981.

Leavitt, Judith Walzer. *Typhoid Mary: Captive to the Public's Health.* Boston: Beacon Press, 1996.

Leviatin, David. "Part One Introduction: Framing the Poor—The Irresistibility of *How the Other Half Lives*." In Jacob A. Riis, editor, *How the Other Half Lives*. Boston: Bedford Books/St. Martin's Press, 2011.

Libster, Martha M. *Herbal Diplomats*. Neenah, WI: Golden Apple Publications, 2004.

Lindenmeyer, Kriste. *"A Right to Childhood": The U.S. Children's Bureau and Child Welfare, 1912–1946*. Urbana: University of Illinois Press, 1997.

Lindsey, Gordon. *John Alexander Dowie: A Life Story of Trials, Tragedies and Triumphs*. Shreveport, LA: Voice of Healing Publishing, 1951.

MacGarvie, Mark Douglas. *Law and Religion in American History: Public Values and Private Conscience*. New York: Cambridge University Press, 2016.

Madden, Deborah. *"A Cheap, Safe, and Natural Medicine": Religion, Medicine, and Culture in John Wesley's "Primitive Physic."* Amsterdam, The Netherlands: Rodopi Press, 2007.

Manseau, Peter. *The Apparitionists*. Boston: Houghton Mifflin, 2017.

Markel, Howard. "For the Welfare of Children: The Origins of the Relationship Between U.S. Public Health Workers and Pediatricians." In Alexandra Minna Stern and Howard Markel, editors, *Formative Years: Children's Health in the United States, 1880–1902*. Ann Arbor, MI: University of Michigan Press, 2004, 47–65.

Mason, Mary Ann. *From Father's Property to Children's Rights: The History of Child Custody in the United States*. New York: Columbia University Press, 1994.

Meckel, Richard A. *Save the Babies: American Public Health Reform and the Prevention of Infant Mortality, 1850–1929*. Baltimore: Johns Hopkins University Press, 1990.

Mintz, Steven. *Huck's Raft: A History of American Childhood*. Cambridge, MA: Harvard University Press, 2006.

Mnookin, Robert H., and D. Kelly Weisberg. *Child, Family, and State: Problems and Materials on Children in the Law*. New York: Aspen Publishers, 2000.

Mohr, James C. *Licensed to Practice: The Supreme Court Defines the American Medical Profession*. Baltimore: Johns Hopkins University Press, 2013.

Morantz-Sanchez, Regina. *Sympathy and Science: Women Physicians in American Medicine*. Reprinted. Chapel Hill, NC: University of North Carolina Press, 2000.

Murray, John E. "Bound by Charity: The Abandoned Children of Late Eighteenth-Century Charleston." In Billy G. Smith, editor, *Down and Out in Early America*. University Park, PA: Pennsylvania State University Press, 2004.

Nelson, Shirley. *Fair, Clear, and Terrible: The Story of Shiloh*. Eugene, OR: Wipf and Stock, 2009.

New York Society for the Prevention of Cruelty to Children. "History." https://www.nyspcc.org/about-the-new-york-society-for-the-prevention-of-cruelty-to-children/history/.

New York State Supreme Court, Historical Society of the New York Courts. http://www.nycourts.gov/history/legal-history-new-york/history-legal-bench-supreme-court.html.

Numbers, Ronald L. *Prophetess of Health: A Study of Ellen G. White.* Third edition. Grand Rapids, MI: William B. Eerdmans Publishing Company, 2008.

Offit, Paul. *Bad Faith: When Religious Belief Undermines Modern Medicine.* New York: Basic Books, 2015.

Opp, James. *The Lord for the Body: Religion, Medicine, and Protestant Faith Healing in Canada, 1880–1930.* Montreal: McGill-Queen's University Press, 2005.

Parish, H. J. *A History of Immunization.* Edinburgh, UK: E and S. Livingstone, 1965.

Pearson, Susan J. *The Rights of the Defenseless: Protecting Animals and Children in Gilded Age America.* Chicago: University of Chicago Press, 2011.

Peters, Shawn Francis. *When Prayer Fails: Faith Healing, Children, and the Law.* New York: Oxford University Press, 2008.

Pleck, Elizabeth. *Domestic Tyranny: The Making of American Social Policy Against Family Violence from Colonial Times to the Present.* New York: Oxford University Press, 1987.

Poloma, Margaret M. "A Comparison of Christian Science and Mainline Christian Healing Ideologies and Practices," *Review of Religious Research,* Volume 32, Number 4 (June 1991): 337–350.

Porter, Roy. *Flesh in the Age of Reason: The Modern Foundations of Body and Soul.* New York: W.W. Norton, 2003.

Porterfield, Amanda. *Healing in the History of Christianity.* New York: Oxford University Press, 2005.

Preston, Samuel H., and Michael R. Haines. *Fatal Years: Child Mortality in Late Nineteenth-Century America.* Princeton, NJ: Princeton University Press, 1991.

Radbill, Samuel. "The Pediatrics of Benjamin Rush," *Transactions and Studies of the College of Physicians of Philadelphia,* Volume 40, Number 3 (January 1973): 151–170.

Robertson, Stephen. *Crimes Against Children: Sexual Violence and Legal Culture in New York City, 1880–1960.* Chapel Hill, NC: University of North Carolina Press, 2005.

Rogers, Alan Rogers. *The Child Cases: How America's Religious Exemption Laws Harm Children.* Amherst: University of Massachusetts Press, 2014.

Rogers, Naomi. "Women and Sectarian Medicine." In Rima D. Apple, editor, *Women, Health, and Medicine in America: A Historical Handbook.* New Brunswick, NJ: Rutgers University Press, 1992.

———. *Dirt and Disease: Polio Before FDR.* New Brunswick, NJ: Rutgers University Press, 1992.

Rosen, George. *A History of Public Health.* Revised expanded edition. Baltimore: Johns Hopkins University Press, 2015.

Rosenberg, Charles E. "The Therapeutic Revolution: Medicine, Meaning, and Social Change in Nineteenth-Century America." In Morris J. Vogel and Charles E. Rosenberg, editors, *The Therapeutic Revolution: Essays in the Social History of American Medicine*. Philadelphia: University of Pennsylvania Press, 1979.

———. "Health in the Home: A Tradition of Print and Practice." In Charles E. Rosenberg, editor, *Right Living: An Angle-American Tradition of Self-Help Medicine and Hygiene*. Baltimore: Johns Hopkins University Press, 2003.

Rothman, David J. *The Discovery of the Asylum: Social Order and Disorder in the New Republic*. New York: Little, Brown, and Company, 1990.

Rothstein, William G. "The Botanical Movements and Orthodox Medicine." In Norman Gevitz, editor, *Other Healers: Unorthodox Medicine in America*. Baltimore: Johns Hopkins University Press, 1988, 29–51.

Sappol, Michael. *A Traffic of Dead Bodies: Anatomy and Embodied Social Identity in Nineteenth-Century America*. Princeton, NJ: Princeton University Press, 2002.

Satter, Beryl. *Each Mind a Kingdom: American Women, Sexual Purity, and the New Thought Movement, 1875-1920*. Berkeley, CA: University of California Press, 1999.

Schmidt, James D. "'Restless Movements Characteristic of Childhood': The Legal Construction of Child Labor in Nineteenth-Century Massachusetts," *Law and History Review*, Volume 23, Number 2 (Summer 2005): 315–350.

———. *Industrial Violence and the Legal Origins of Child Labor*. New York: Cambridge University Press, 2010.

Schmidt, William H. "Health and Welfare of Colonial American Children," *American Journal of Diseases of Children*, Volume 130 (July 1976): 694–670.

Schoepflin, Rennie B. *Christian Science on Trial: Religious Healing on Trial*. Baltimore: Johns Hopkins University Press, 2003.

Sealander, Judith. *The Failed Century of the Child: Governing America's Young in the Twentieth Century*. New York: Cambridge University Press, 2003.

Shelman, Eric A., and Stephen Lazoritz, editors. *The Mary Ellen Wilson Child Abuse Case and the Beginning of Children's Rights in 19th Century America*. Jefferson, NC: McFarland and Company, 2005.

Shryock, Richard Harrison. *Medicine and Society in America 1660–1860*. New York: New York University Press, 1960.

———. *Medical Licensing in America, 1650–1965*. Baltimore: Johns Hopkins University Press, 1967.

Stark, Rodney. "The Rise and Fall of Christian Science," *Journal of Contemporary Religion*, Volume 13, Number 2 (1998): 189–214.

Starr, Paul. *The Social Transformation of American Medicine*. New York: Basic Books, 1982.

Steedman, Carolyn. *Strange Dislocations: Childhood and the Idea of Human Interiority, 1789–1830*. Cambridge, MA: Harvard University Press, 1995.

Steenburg, Nancy Hathaway. *Children and the Criminal Law in Connecticut, 1635–1855: Changing Perceptions of Childhood*. New York: Routledge, 2005.

Stern, Alexandra Minna, and Howard Markel, editors. "Introduction." In *Formative Years: Children's Health in the United States, 1880–2000*. Ann Arbor: University of Michigan Press, 2004, 1–20.

Swan, Rita. "On Statutes Depriving a Class of Children of Rights to Medical Care: Can This Discrimination Be Litigated?" *Quinnipiac Health Law Journal*, Volume 2, Number 73 (1998).

Tanenhaus, David S. "Between Dependency and Liberty: The Conundrum of Children's Rights in the Gilded Age," *Law and History Review*, Volume 23, Number 2 (Summer 2005): 351–385.

"The 1901 St. Louis Incident: The First Modern Medical Disaster," *Pediatrics*, Volume 133, Issue 6 (June 2014): 964–965.

Trescher, Robert L., and Thomas N. O'Neill, Jr. "Medical Care for Dependent Children: Manslaughter Liability of the Christian Scientist," *University of Pennsylvania Law Review*, Volume 109 (1960): 203–217.

Truax, Rhonda. *The Doctors Jacobi*. Boston: Little, Brown, and Company, 1952.

Viner, Russell. "Abraham Jacobi and the Origins of Scientific Pediatrics in America." In Alexandra Minna Stern and Howard Markel, editors, *Formative Years: Children's Health in the United States, 1880–2000*. Ann Arbor, MI: University of Michigan Press, 2004, 23–46.

Wacker, Grant. "Marching to Zion: Religion in a Modern Utopian Community," *Church History*, Volume 54, Number 4 (December 1985): 496–511.

Walloch, Karen L. *The Antivaccine Heresy: Jacobson v. Massachusetts and the Troubled History of Compulsory Vaccination in the United States*. Rochester, NY: University of Rochester Press, 2015.

Wardell, Walter I. "Christian Science Healing," *Journal for the Scientific Study of Religion*, Volume 4, Number 2 (Spring 1965): 171–181.

Watson, Katherine D. *Forensic Medicine in Western Society: A History*. New York: Routledge, 2011.

Weindling, Paul. "From Research to Clinical Practice: Serum Therapy for Diphtheria in the 1890s. In John V. Pickstone, editor, *Medical Innovations in Historical Perspective*. New York: St. Martin's Press, 1992, 72–83.

Whooley, Owen. *Knowledge in the Time of Cholera*. Chicago: University of Chicago Press, 2013.

Whorton, James C. *Nature Cures: The History of Alternative Medicine in America*. Oxford University Press, 2002.

Williams, Joseph W. *Spirit Cure: A History of Pentecostal Healing*. New York: Oxford University Press, 2013.

Willrich, Michael C. *Pox: An American History*. New York: Penguin, 2011.

Wilson, Brian C., Dr. *John Harvey Kellogg and the Religion of Biologic Living*. Bloomington, IN: Indiana University Press, 2014.

Winter, Allison. *Mesmerized: Powers of Mind in Victorian Britain*. Chicago: University of Chicago Press, 1998.

Woodhouse, Barbara Bennett. *Hidden in Plain Sight: The Tragedy of Children's Rights from Ben Franklin to Lionel Tate*. Princeton, NJ: Princeton University Press, 2008.

Zelizer, Vivian A. *Pricing the Priceless Child: The Changing Social Value of Children*. New York: Basic Books, 1985.

Zion Historical Society. *Zion*. Charleston, SC: Arcadia Publishing, 2007.

Ziporyn, Terra. *Disease in the Popular Press: The Case of Diphtheria, Typhoid Fever, and Syphilis, 1870–1920*. New York: Greenwood Press, 1988.

# Index

The manufacturer's authorised representative in the EU is Springer
Nature Customer Service Centre GmbH, Europaplatz 3, 69115 Heidelberg,
Germany. If you have any concerns regarding our products, please
contact ProductSafety@springernature.com

Printed and bound by CPI Group (UK) Ltd, Croydon, CR0 4YY
29/04/2026
02099458-0001